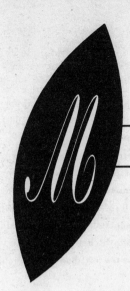

M ISCONCEPTIONS

THE SOCIAL
CONSTRUCTION
OF CHOICE AND
THE NEW
REPRODUCTIVE
AND GENETIC
TECHNOLOGIES

**VOLUME
ONE**

EDITORS

**GWYNNE BASEN • MARGRIT EICHLER
ABBY LIPPMAN**

Publishing Editor: Sean Fordyce

82 Frontenac Street, Hull, Quebec J8X 1Z5 (819) 778-2946

Cover design: Beth Haliburton/Loco Design

Book Interior design: Sean Fordyce and Beth Haliburton

First Edition (Volume One) November, 1993.

Canadian Cataloguing in Publication Data:

   Misconceptions: the social construction of choice and the new reproductive and genetic technologies

Includes bibliographical references.

ISBN 0-921842-25-2 (v. 1) -

ISBN 0-921842-37-6 (v. 2)

   1. Human reproductive technology. 2. Human reproductive technology — Social aspects.

I. Basen, Gwynne. II. Eichler, Margrit. III. Lippman, Abby.

RG133.5.M48 1993   326.1'98178   C94-900017-5

Printed in Canada by Webcom Ltd., Toronto.

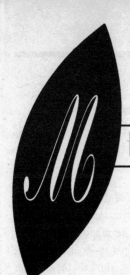

MISCONCEPTIONS

THE SOCIAL
CONSTRUCTION
OF CHOICE AND
THE NEW
REPRODUCTIVE
AND GENETIC
TECHNOLOGIES

VOLUME ONE

EDITORS

**GWYNNE BASEN • MARGRIT EICHLER
ABBY LIPPMAN**

82 FRONTENAC STREET,
HULL, QUEBEC J8X 1Z5

TEL: |819| 778-2946
FAX: |819| 778-2940

VOYAGEUR   PUBLISHING

ACKNOWLEDGMENTS

The editors and publishers of this book would like to acknowledge the contribution of Mount Saint Vincent University through the support afforded by the Nancy Rowell Jackman Chair in Women's Studies at the Mount to Margrit Eichler, who held the Chair in 1992-93. This allowed us to translate the French language materials into English.

Special thanks to Vanessa Hill for the very many ways in which she kept the book (and the editors) moving along; to Leopold Plotek for his support and assistance; and to friends and families who, in innumerable ways, participated in and contributed to the conception, gestation and "delivery" of this book.

CONTRIBUTORS

EDITORS
GWYNNE BASEN MARGRIT EICHLER
ABBY LIPPMAN

CONTRIBUTING AUTHORS

Rosanna Baraldi	Abby Lippman
Maria Barile	Maggie MacDonald
Gwynne Basen	Christine Massey
Ronda Bessner	Heather Menzies
Annette Burfoot	Karen Messing
Varda Burstyn	Lisa M. Mitchell
Karen Capen	Gail Ouellette
Gena Corea	Judy Rebick
Lynda Davies	Susan Sherwin
Margrit Eichler	Harriet Simand
Kate Fillion	Laura Sky
Lynn Glazier	Sunera Thobani
Sandra A. Goundry	Sari Tudiver
Donna Launslager	Louise Vandelac

Translation of Articles Received In
French by Sheila Fischman

TABLE OF CONTENTS VOLUME I

PART I: SETTING THE CONTEXT

PART II: EUGENICS: FROM THEN TO NOW

PART III: THE ROYAL COMMISSION ON NEW REPRODUCTIVE TECHNOLOGIES: A COSTLY FAILURE?

TABLE OF CONTENTS VOLUME II

PART V: WOMEN AS GESTATORS; CHILDREN AS PRODUCTS

PART VI: PUBLIC POLICIES

We are all daughters although we may not all be mothers. We offer this book in the hope that it will help insure true and full procreative freedom for future generations.

GWYNNE BASEN
MARGRIT EICHLER
ABBY LIPPMAN

This book is one of two volumes that emerged from a collaborative effort between the editors and the individual authors. This collaboration is reflected in the alphabetical listing of the editors as well as in the generous participation of the 26 women who wrote most of the words that follow under extraordinary time and resource constraints imposed by their already overcommitted schedules. Any profits from royalties will go to the NAC Charitable and Educational Trust.

We have long been troubled by the Royal Commission and as the date for release of its report seemed to be getting closer, we felt we had to do something about our concerns: something that would open consideration of the new reproductive and genetic technologies beyond the "official" word to come from the Commission. Something that would keep the discussion open and participatory. This collection is a first step to open the issues.

The papers in this book do not speak for all women. Most important, we as editors and writers of chapters do not — and would not want to — *presume* to speak for all women.

What we offer, rather, are some voices. We asked women whose views we wanted to read and to share with others to join us. (And we apologize to those who are missing because space and time limits, theirs and ours, precluded the contributions we would have liked from them.) To the ear, some may seem political, some personal, some polemical. They are all of these, and more. They are the uneven, untranslated voices of women who represent themselves and no one else. We have encouraged this diversity, aiming not for an academic monotone but for an accessible *a capella* chorus.

Thus, the voices here speak at many levels, with many sounds. But the chorus is incomplete; many other voices need to be heard. Perhaps the sounds of concern, anger and pain expressed here will encourage the public not only to begin listening carefully to what we are told about the new reproductive and genetic technologies but also to raise their voices with us.

INTRODUCTION: FIRST WORDS

Gena Corea

An elderly couple walk among the physicians and scientists in the lobby of the Hilton Hotel Convention Centre in Jerusalem in 1989 silently handing to each "technodoc" a photocopy of a letter they have written. The couple are afraid. Would these participants of the Sixth World Congress on In Vitro Fertilization and Alternate Assisted Reproduction call the police? Throw them out? That prospect was terrifying yet, as the old man, Alexander Werba, 67, told me, that was actually — when he later thought about it — what he wanted: he wanted the police to scream in with sirens, and reporters to rush in with them, notebooks open, cameras rolling, and then he could tell them why he and his wife had come, how these doctors — no, they were no doctors, he said angrily, they were child-production engineers — how they had killed his daughter.

Alexander is white-haired, round and short, with bushy white eyebrows protruding from the glasses that cover his blue eyes. His wife, Prima, 61, is small, thin, her black hair streaked in grey, her glasses hanging from a cord. Both wear white sneakers. I watch them weave among the tall, fit, well-dressed technodocs who are drinking coffee and chatting in small groups on a break during the Congress.

The letter the Werbas distribute states that their daughter, Aliza Eisenberg, died as a result of an egg capture procedure in the *in vitro* fertilization (IVF) program at Haddassah Hospital and protests the fact that the physician who performed that egg capture had been named secretary of the Congress.

"Mein Herz klopft so," Prima whispers to me as she passes quickly by me. ("My heart is beating so.")

I had spoken with the couple for hours the night before about the death of their daughter and they had shown me the letter they planned to pass out this morning at the Congress. They had come to Jerusalem from Haifa in order to do it.

They speak no English and fear that if a technodoc reading the letter addresses them, they will be unable to understand or reply.

Prima approaches the huge lecture hall to which the technodocs will soon return. She tries to enter but a woman in the red uniform of the congress employees stops her. Prima is not registered for the congress. She has no badge.

Fearing the uniformed woman, Prima waits until she leaves. Then she enters the hall, empty of physicians, and places a letter on each of the seats, always looking to each side to see that no one is coming.

As she is leaving, she looks up, spots a young man, catches a glimpse of the name on his badge: It's him! The man who took her daughter's eggs. The man who left her daughter bleeding to death.

Prima quickly exits. She and Alexander are too upset, too frightened, to continue distributing the letter. Trembling, they leave the convention centre.

* * * * *

The Werbas' fear went deeper than a concern that they wouldn't be able to understand the technodocs' English. They explained it to me later when I visited them in their home in Haifa.

Poles, they both survived the Nazi time in Europe. Alexander's parents had been transported in a train to Treblinka. After running away from a work camp and obtaining false identity papers, he lived on the Aryan side of Warsaw, working in the darkroom of a photography shop, thankful he did not have to be out in the dangerous streets. He was afraid all the time. The fear he had felt during that year and a half in Warsaw, before he joined the resistance, was exactly the fear he felt at the IVF Congress, he told me.

Prima's family had been loaded onto a cargo train that would end at the crematorium in Belzec, Poland. Her father and brother died there. Her grandmother told the 14-year-old Prima to jump from the train. She did. Living for 15 months in hay in the attic of a good woman, she survived the war. She still dreams of that time.

"She dreams that the Germans are running and shooting," Alexander tells me. "Soldiers and SS men. She sees that in her dreams very often. Now, after this case with our daughter, she dreams more often about doctors. Every night."

She told me of her reaction to seeing for the first time the man who had attempted IVF on her daughter. "I was afraid like when I was with the Germans, when they led me to the crematorium in the cargo train."

"There were many people from the conference centre to make sure that everything was in order and was going 100 percent smoothly," Alexander explains, "and she saw the Nazis in every such official in the red uniforms. All these associations. Maybe they would throw us out. Or arrest us. You understand me? I didn't want it to come to that. But now I am sorry I didn't make a big scene where they called the police and arrested me or tried to throw me out. Then someone would have come from the press or television and I could have said in the press everything that was written in the letter. But at that time I was so — that was dumb. They were no Germans. Why was I so afraid? I wanted to go sit in a corner where no one could see me."

* * * * *

The association Prima and Alexander made between life under the Nazis and their daughter's ordeal from the reproductive technology experimentation is an association consciously made by several women writing in this vital book.

Lynn Glazier recognizes in the new reproductive technologies the totalitarian project of controlling who will be allowed to be born into this world; the eugenic attempt to eradicate, even before birth, the lives of those judged "unworthy of life."

She points out that the Nazis' "Final Solution" originated in mainstream medicine; that more than 70,000 people — patients all — were killed in gas chambers installed in hospitals — psychiatric hospitals; that the doctors and gas chambers were then moved to Poland to kill ("heal," in the Nazi metaphor) on a grander scale; and that the Nazis called this "the great therapy of Auschwitz."

Varda Burstyn discusses the special responsibility many Germans today feel to speak out against and stop the proliferation of new reproductive technologies (NRTs) because they well understand what is going on here and where it leads.

She refers to the first international feminist conference in resistance to the new reproductive technologies held in Bonn in 1985. Her mention of it brought memories alive, for I addressed that conference. One such memory: a young woman in jeans, Theresia Degener, delivers a paper to a speaker on stage. She holds the paper in her teeth. She has no arms. She had not been injured by genes. (As several authors in this volume, including Sandra Goundry, point out, genes are responsible for a small portion — 3 to 5 percent — of disabilities.) No. She had been injured by medical treatment, in the form of Thalidomide, administered by well-educated, mainstream physicians.

The first time I met Theresia, in Frankfurt, Germany, she interviewed me for a magazine article. With her toe, she turned her tape-recorder on and when the recorder malfunctioned, she impatiently pushed it aside with one foot, pulled a pen and notebook out from her tote bag, again with a foot, and, as I spoke, scribbled notes with the pen between two toes.

In the following years, we often worked together at conferences of the Feminist International Network of Resistance to Reproductive and Genetic Engineering (FINRRAGE). At one such conference in Mallorca, Spain, I remember her laughter, her exuberance. She told me at breakfast that she'd worked much of the night on the paper she was to give that afternoon. She hadn't wanted to disturb her roommate's sleep so she brought her typewriter to the hall outside her hotel room and typed there, with her feet. Several people had staggered down the hall drunk at 3 a.m. and she could just imagine them now at breakfast, she told me, her eyes sparkling in delight, saying they were so drunk last night they thought they saw an armless woman in the hall typing with her feet! We roared laughing.

One afternoon on Mallorca, I rounded a bend in the road and the sea suddenly appeared far below me and there was Theresia standing on a rock. In the next moment, she leapt and dove head first — an armless dive — into the sea. The sight of her — joyous and courageous — took my breath away.

A few years later, Theresia and a paralyzed friend in a wheelchair traveled together in the U.S. I met the two women in Boston several times for dinner. In restaurant restrooms, while I washed my hands before the meal, Theresia washed her feet. At the table, she would wield her fork between her toes, her foot reaching from the plate to her mouth.

This quickly became so normal to me that I was sometimes startled when a waiter, after bringing our dinners, stayed by the table staring at Theresia. Annoyed at his interrupting the flow of our conversation, I'd puzzle for a second: What's he staring at?

But before eating with fork between toes did become natural to me, Theresia made me look anew at my feet. I had thought of them as just ends of something. Something that walked, ran. Not much more. What a failure of imagination I routinely practiced — using my feet merely to walk. How infinite were their possibilities! How I'd undervalued them. I'd looked at them all these years and not truly seen them. My body was more fascinating, more capable than I had ever imagined and I was not living my body as fully as Theresia showed a body could be lived.

Imagine Theresia, with her empathy for others, her courage, her creativity, her determination, her intelligence, her joy — all qualities she took to law school with her, all qualities that infuse her work in the disability rights movement in Germany and in the international feminist movement of resistance to reproductive and genetic engineering — imagine Theresia, on some prenatal test, judged "life unworthy of life!"

Take special care in reading the fine chapters in this book that challenge the fascist project of eliminating "unworthy" life (like Theresia's!) through use of the new reproductive technologies. Abby Lippman's chapter poses vital questions that Theresia Degener would also ask: "Why have efforts to find every fetus with Down syndrome become so important to us that universal triple screening is entering recommended medical practice, while ensuring early prenatal care for all women (the lack of which is a major cause of disability) is still an unachieved goal?"

*****

Gwynne Basen and Heather Menzies refer in their chapters to the fact that it's not only reproduction that is now being engineered. The public discussion of the NRTs and of genetic engineering is also engineered. The forces behind medicine and industry have been largely successful in controlling the kind of information and the kind of interpretation ("stories," in Abby Lippman's insightful phrasing) we receive on the technologies.

The public discussion, Basen notes, is "framed in a way that excluded any consideration of the risks or ethical considerations."

What's left out of the framework is just what the authors of *Misconceptions* insist on including in the alternative framework they provide: the extraordinarily high failure rate of IVF; the experimental nature of the techniques; the damage of the techniques to women physically, emotionally and spiritually; the preventable and ignored causes of infertility — including environmental factors (see chapter by Karen Messing and Gail Ouellette) and sexually transmitted diseases — some of those diseases, as Lynda Davies points out in a crucial chapter, transmitted to the women when they were sexually abused as children; increasing medical and technological control over procreation (Ronda Bessner and most other chapters); the violations of women's integrity, dignity and freedom involved in the techniques (see, for example, Kate Fillion and the chapters on commissioned pregnancies by Margrit Eichler and Susan Sherwin); the unimaginable stress placed on women who suddenly become the mothers of three or four infants following the implantation of multiple embryos (see the chapter by Donna Launslager with Ulla Colgrass); the increasing industrialization of reproduction (see chapters by Sari Tudiver and Gwynne Basen); woman's status in a sexual caste system (see chapter by Sunera Thobani); the increasing use of women as experimental models for other species (see Annette Burfoot's chapter).

When ethics are publically discussed, women's experiences are largely absent from consideration. At the IVF congress in Jerusalem where the Werbas passed out their letter, the panel on ethics was entirely composed of men. The men did not notice the omission of women. It occurred to none of them that experimentation on women might be an ethical issue related to IVF. No one spoke of the Nuremberg or Helsinki codes on protection of human experimental subjects, let alone pointed out the many ways IVF violates those codes. (And IVF *is* experimentation as feminist analyses have been documenting for years and as the World Health Organization has acknowledged.) Though the moderator of the ethics panel was on the IVF team at Haddassah Hospital, Aliza Eisenberg's name never passed his lips.

The reproduction industry's control of the public discussion of the new reproductive technologies in the U.S. is just as complete as it is in Britain. Canadians have fine films critically examining the NRTs: *On the Eighth Day: Perfecting Mother Nature. Part One: Making Babies. Part Two: Making Perfect Babies.* We in the United States have nothing comparable. The technodocs are in complete control of the public discussion.

In Canada, The Royal Commission on New Reproduction Technologies has been designated as a major framer of the public discussion of the technologies. Many principled women, seeing the enormous impact these technologies would have on the lives of all generations of women to come, devoted two years of their lives to lobbying for the establishment of this commission, believing that through the commission, the truth would out.

The betrayal of these women, and all women, is documented in enraging detail in Part III of this book. As these papers make clear, the public discussion of reproductive engineering is being engineered.

* * * * *

Gwynne Basen writes that as she listens to an IVF doc tell her that in 50 years, there will be no relationship between sex and human procreation, she knows that it is for her young daughter that she is working to oppose the proliferation of the new reproductive technologies.

I feel her same sense of protection towards the women who will be born (or extracted) after us. Basen's comment brought this memory to my consciousness and, with it, a compelling desire that many more women join us in safeguarding the future generation of daughters.

I interviewed a technodoc in her IVF clinic outside Paris in 1988, asking questions about the new experimental method of superovulating women: the administration of analogues, drugs that cut off the brain's control of the ovary so that doctors, through their administration of hormones, can take over that control. Technodocs were saying of Buserline, the trade name for an analogue commonly used in France, that it "cuts the high command." One technodoc called it "physiological decapitation." Another had described Buserline as causing a chemical menopause, but the woman I am interviewing disagrees with this.

"It's more like a woman without a head," she tells me evenly.

"Excuse me?"

The drug cuts off the connection between the woman's head and her ovary, she explains, so it's like a woman without a head.

She sees no problem at all with this.

After the interview, she offers me a ride back to the city. It is raining torrentially. As the windshield wipers squeak back and forth, she mentions that she and a colleague on the IVF team sometimes bring their young daughters to the hospital with them on a Saturday when they have work to do and the girls play test-tube baby in the lab. The children take a test-tube, fill it with water and pretend that a bubble in the water is the baby. She smiles indulgently, as if telling an endearing story.

I keep my voice normal though I am chilled at the thought of little girls growing up, never having known a world without laboratory reproduction. "To the girls being born now," I comment, my voice a false neutral, "all this will seem completely normal and everyday."

"Yes, yes, completely normal."

She tells me that she has talked with her five-year-old child about birth and because she thought the child was too young to understand vaginal birth, she explained cesarean sections to her. Sometimes, she says, her daughter plays at having a baby by taking a knife and running it across her doll's stomach.

Maybe, I think, as the windshield wipers squeak in the Parisian rain, she could play IVF by chopping off her doll's head.

*****

During that week in Paris conducting interviews, I became filled with horror at what was going on. In that week alone, I learned of four more deaths of women in IVF programs. (I know of 16 now, surely not the full toll, since the technodocs have taken care to provide no mechanism for collecting information on serious accidents and deaths from IVF, and I have learned what I know only by pursuing isolated leaks.)

At the end of this week, I sat at a party with Louise Vandelac, an internationally known analyst of the NRTs, one of the four commissioners fired from the Royal Commission on New Reproductive Technologies, and a contributor to this volume. I spoke inarticulately of my horror at women dying namelessly, without record or notice; my horror at the pornographic woman-without-a-head. (Someone, discussing the analogue method of superovulation, had joked grimly at the party earlier, "After cutting off the woman's head, they ask for informed consent.")

"I feel a growing terror in the pit of my stomach when I see people's reactions to it all," I tell Louise. "They don't see anything wrong. It's all very normal to them."

I mention a lunch we had both had this week with Dr. Sacha Geller, who ran a contractual pregnancy firm in Marseilles and whom I had debated at a public forum. (Contractual pregnancy was widely called "surrogate motherhood" back then, a term Margrit Eichler wisely refuses to adopt.)

During the lunch, I reminded Louise, I told Geller about Denise Mounce, the young woman who died while carrying a pregnancy under contract with a reproduction company in the U.S. I asked him if that would change the way he viewed contractual pregnancies. He had looked at me blankly for a moment and then said:

"But we have insurance."

"Oh," I'd said, stunned. "Then it's not a problem? That solves the problem?"

"Yes," he's replied, "That solves the problem."

Nodding in grim remembrance, Louise responds: "The worst is yet to come. These deaths are just the beginning. It's like the 1930s now. We know how some people in the 30s must have felt, smelling what was to come. These are pre-fascist times."

Misconceptions is a book by women who can smell it coming. It's a demanding book because once you smell it too, you have to take some action in the world to stop it. It's our human duty to ourselves, to our own dignity, to our souls.

PART I

SETTING THE CONTEXT

"It's so distressing, I can't conceive at all"; "It's so overwhelming, I can't conceive of it all." Two women speak. Their words are slightly different, but their two voices merge. Women conceive babies; women conceive ideas. We have conceptions of all sorts — some made of flesh and blood and others only in our minds. How easily the term adapts to both usages.

Misconceptions, the title of this volume, is another word with two layers of meaning, layers that are stripped off for analysis in the chapters in this section. And there is a further echo in the word if one lets an additional sound enter because then it speaks of what is claimed to have focused attention on this area in the first place: "missed conceptions," the pregnancies and children that women wanted or expected to have that did not occur on time, or at all. (And maybe, too, the conceptions that will be missed as production makes procreation a relic of the past.)

Misconceptions about ideas/words and (mis)conceptions of children surround us in this age of the new reproductive and genetic technologies. And how dangerous the misconceptions — of both sorts — are. Physicians speak of "products of conception," the embryos and fetuses nurtured by a woman during her pregnancy, while feminists worry about making conception a consumer good, a product. Experimentation is conceived and promoted (by physicians) as "treatment"; manipulation — of eggs, embryos, the genetic material itself, and, most centrally, women — is conceived and promoted (again by physicians and the biomedical professionals) as "care" and "cure." Conceptions become products, human and intellectual, leading to misconceptions of deed and of thought that are entangled as one leads to the other in a pernicious cycle.

These are the issues these introductory chapters seek to unravel and trace. Unravel, so that the interlocking threads that blend reproductive with genetic technologies into the whole cloth of today's human reproduction can be seen; trace, so that the technologies can be exposed as part of a single Möbius strip, the same side of a troublesome reality in which women's desires for (healthy) children become the justification for creating profits and experimental objects, for using one human as the means to the ends of another.

Words have been used by biomedicine to sell the new reproductive and genetic technologies: GIFTs,* BABIs,* surrogates** distance us from what is occurring. The authors in this section speak to reclaiming words, to reclaiming power and to redefining the paradigm within which we conceive of reproduction and within which we reproduce.

It is the "one-ness" of these technologies that the chapters here and elsewhere in the book emphasize. Body parts, whole persons, now the human genome itself — all are commercial property. Pregnancy is business, big business, and in business the best product is the most profitable one. Quality is sold, with quality depending on the production of certain embryos, on allowing only selected fetuses to be born and certain women to give birth. Cost-benefit ratios are calculated in biomedical terms to advance the sales pitch for technology use. There is "one-ness" not only of the biotechnologies themselves, where there is no pre-implantation diagnosis without embryo transfer, no contract mothers without mandatory prenatal diagnosis, no genetic manipulation without "spare" embryos and frozen eggs, but also of their repercussions for women's lives and health, in Canada and worldwide: control, marginalization and victimization. As Sari Tudiver and Abby Lippman demonstrate, whether they be to prevent, create or monitor conception, the genetic technologies and reproductive technologies come from the same agenda, with their internationalization and commercialization making them global concerns.

Kafka is a name that recurs in this book, usually paired with the Royal Commission to evoke the state of senseless oppression of Joseph K in *The Trial.* But this author's name evokes another image, one that especially resonates throughout the chapters in this section: an image of metamorphosis. Changes are depicted by all the authors, fundamental changes in how we conceive new life and changes in how we conceive of new lives and the technologies that create them. This is especially transparent in the paper by Gwynne Basen which describes vividly the power of the technologies as agents of change.

Conception, as it occurs today, has itself been transformed at the same time as it is transforming our values and beliefs. These initial chapters provide an overview and critique of these transformations. They make clear why we must think of the reproductive and genetic technologies not as ways for providing conceptions to respond to the "needs" and "desires" of women but rather as orchestrated misconceptions that in fact subvert these very needs and desires and sabotage the development of long-term, women-centered solutions to women's very real problems.

*See chapters by Basen and Lippman for definition

**See chapters by Eichler and Sherwin for definition

1

FOLLOWING FRANKENSTEIN: WOMEN, TECHNOLOGY AND THE FUTURE OF PROCREATION

Gwynne Basen

"A new species would bless me as its creator and source; many happy and excellent natures would owe their being to me. No father could claim the gratitude of his child so completely as I should deserve theirs."

Mary Shelley,
"Frankenstein"

"I gave the little eggs names. I had already attributed a personality to them, feminine of course... I invested myself in a role that was not paternal. I felt I was the lover, not the father."

Jacques Testart,
IVF scientist and critic.

The reproductive technologies currently employed in clinics around the world may be new — or as one IVF doctor pointed out to me, new as applied to women, since they have been in use in the cattle barns for a long time — but there is nothing new about the social relations from which they have emerged. Inequalities of gender, class and race are deeply embedded in the operating programs of the technologies. As technology begins to assume a larger and larger role in procreation, those doctors, scientists, lawyers, politicians and ethicists who create and control these techniques and monitor their use will decide who will have children, when and how. The more these reproductive technologies become the property of private commercial interests, the more the business of baby-making will be restricted to those who can pay for it.

The scientific-commercial interests behind the rapid expansion of the reproductive technologies have also been largely successful in controlling the kind of information we receive about them. Each new scientific "triumph" has been dutifully reported by the media — whether it be the first babies born from frozen embryos, or the latest set of IVF quintuplets. In American newspapers and magazines, advertisements for fertility clinics feature photographs of cherubic newborns and call out to infertile couples, "Before you let go of the dream, talk to us." What we don't find in these newspaper headlines and advertisements are the controversies and the conflicts that are as much a part of IVF and the other new reproductive technologies as the glowing reports that reach the public.

Years of research by feminist critics and critical scientists have produced an ever-increasing set of evidence on the multiple risks of these procedures and their troubling consequences. Nonetheless, the low success rates, the experimental nature of the techniques, the increasing medical and technological control over procreation and the links between IVF and genetic manipulation are seldom discussed in the mainstream media.

Typical of the media's approach to this subject is an interview I watched on the CBC noon news show, *Midday*. Ralph Benmergui, the host at that time, was interviewing Dr. Murray Kroach from the Toronto East General Hospital IVF clinic, called the LIFE program. (LIFE — for Laboratory Initiated Fetal Emplacement!) Kroach is also one of the owners of a private clinic in Toronto called IVF Canada. The day before, the first baby in Canada to have begun as a frozen embryo had been born.

Benmergui began by congratulating Kroach and asking him about the procedure. Then he hit him with the big question: did the doctor feel there were any ethical questions raised by this new technology? Kroach's answer was a brief, "No. This was a desperate infertile couple and I gave them a baby."

"Oh, right," said Benmergui, who then moved on to the next question on his list. The interview ends, Benmergui thanks the doctor, turns to us, the audience, and reads the last piece of his script. He tells us that there do seem to be some ethical concerns in freezing embryos. But Benmergui doesn't tell us what they are, and if Kroach knew, he certainly isn't going to let us know.

This is the kind of public discussion we have had about these technologies, a discussion that excludes any consideration of risks, consequences or ethics. Embryo freezing — a technology that is employed to improve the low success rate of IVF, a technology that has created a new category of human life, the frozen or "surplus" embryo — is presented to us without question. Or I guess you could say in this case, without answer.

Gena Corea, author of the ground-breaking book *The Mother Machine*, projects that by the year 2050, "Women will be divorced from their own procreative powers, as we (in our generation) are divorced from our own sexuality... These will be women who from their earliest days, grew up with the reality of IVF, embryo transfer, surrogate motherhood, artificial wombs, and sex predetermination technology. From childhood, these women will have watched television news reports involving the storage authority, that is the board in charge of frozen sperm, eggs and human embryos."[1]

A few years ago I listened to an IVF doctor tell me that fifty years from now there will be no relationship between sex and human procreation. His schedule is a little different from Gena Corea's but the dystopic vision remains the same: a world where reproduction will be "a complicated technical process carried out by highly skilled men who use, as raw material for their achievements, the body parts of a variety of interchangeable females."[2]

As I listened to that doctor I thought of my daughter, whose procreative life will begin in the twenty-first century, and I know that the work I am doing to stop the unquestioned, uncontrolled proliferation of these technologies is for her.

Television is a major source of information, and misinformation, about these new technologies. Recently, news shows have taken a back seat to dramas, as a spate of made-for-T.V. movies have appeared, based on the latest medical "miracle."

One night at a friend's house, the conversation turned to the story of the woman in California who had a baby because she needed a bone marrow donor for an older child who has leukaemia. The story had been the movie of that week. My friend thought the woman's intention was to abort her fetus and use its tissue for the bone marrow transplant. But he had some of the details wrong. In this case they needed a baby, not a fetus, to supply the necessary human parts. It is not surprising that my friend made that mistake, because we have all read about experiments using fetal brain tissue to treat Parkinson disease and other neurological conditions. There is a large research effort at Dalhousie University in Halifax that is involved with fetal tissue experiments.

A few years ago, I read two articles about these procedures that appeared on the same day in the *Globe and Mail*. They provided a classic example of how information is presented to us in an utterly fragmented fashion. The first article, on the front page, reported on the Dalhousie Project. According to the article, the only ethical questions raised about this work came from those in the anti-choice movement concerned with the possibility of what they called "fetal harvesting."[3] The other article, on page 9 of the same edition, would seem to have a solution to those concerns. "Within ten years, scientists will have learned how to grow fetal brain tissue in a laboratory dish, thus sidestepping an ethical dilemma facing today's researchers, a Yale University Professor of medicine said yesterday... The researchers also believe that laboratory-grown tissue might in fact be superior candidates for transplantation because their exact point of maturation can be controlled... Tissue culture techniques are liable to defuse the debates over the use of aborted fetal tissue. Once the cells are available, ethical concerns... will become less pressing..."[4]

Once again technology promises to relieve us from any ethical dilemmas. But how? You can only grow, or "culture," fetal tissue from fetuses. This superior laboratory product would still have to come from fetuses, and they would still come from women.

Fetal harvesting is already big business in the United States. One company with the grand name of The International Institute For The Advancement of Medicine, processes over eight thousand fetal parts every year, bringing in close to $1 million in sales.[5] It's a growth industry as fetuses become one of most valuable commodities in biomedical experimentation.

There are markets for other types of human research material as well. As is often the case, these new developments come directly from the livestock industry.

To increase the number of embryos available to them, animal scientists take the ovaries of cows collected from abattoirs, suck out the eggs, mature them in the lab and fertilize them. This technique, called ova *in vitro* maturation, is now used in human reproduction, marketed, of course, as an infertility treatment, even though this industrial-scale production of embryos goes well beyond such a limited use.

An article in the *Boston Globe* describing the first successful efforts at *in vitro* maturation in humans had as its headline, "In Vitro Fertilization Breakthrough."[6] It described the expensive, complex, and uncomfortable processes of IVF and went on to say, "Now women wouldn't need to be subjected to the costly ovarian stimulation drugs, which, while causing harmful side effects, are essential in providing sufficient amounts of mature eggs."[7] Interesting how quick they are to criticize one set of technologies — the use of huge amounts of fertility drugs — when they are out to flog yet another. The piece went on to state that, "At a time when there is an unmet demand for donor eggs by women who cannot produce their own, the Korean research also raises the prospect of establishing 'egg banks' of frozen ova, as is now done routinely with sperm. 'This is an absolutely fantastic result,' said Dr. Martin Quigley of the Cleveland Clinic. 'It could lead to a vast simplification of *in vitro* fertilization,' he told the reporters at the annual meeting of the American Fertility Society."[8]

It is easy to understand Dr. Quigley's enthusiasm. He runs an egg donor program at his Cleveland, Ohio clinic where he has recruited a pool of potential egg "donors" to match to women who are unable or unwilling to use their own eggs. The egg recipients are matched to a suitable donor according to national origin, height, weight, hair colour, eye colour, and blood type, the same kind of matching that is done with donated sperm. The recipient women pay $5,000 U.S. for each *in vitro* attempt. The "donor" women are paid $1,200 for their eggs.

The attempt to successfully freeze human eggs is proving more difficult than first anticipated but there are now several research teams racing to be the first to get it right. When the technology to freeze eggs becomes part of clinical practice, as it will, and egg banks are as common as those for sperm, another technology with the capacity to substantially redefine the origins of human life will have quietly slipped into place, heralded as yet another "breakthrough" in helping the infertile and in expanding women's reproductive choices. Women will have little or no connection to the creation of embryos and the embryo will be reduced to the material status of experimental matter.

Consider how *in vitro* egg maturation and egg freezing can be used to solve the "ethical dilemmas" of using aborted fetal tissue and to expand that area of research. Ovaries can be taken from cadavers or fetuses. Large numbers of eggs can be matured to create a large number of embryos. Currently an embryo will survive in a petri dish until it reaches the stage where it would begin to implant in the uterus. Having nothing to implant into, it begins to flatten out, stops developing and dies. It is hard to get exact information on how long the embryo can be sustained *in vitro*. The outside figure I have heard is 20-30 days, so let's say about three weeks. According to the article in the *Globe and Mail*, those experiments in growing fetal brain tissue use fetuses that are "roughly eight to eleven weeks old."[9] So we are left with a five week gap. For now. In the Reproductive Medicine Unit at the University of Bologna, Italy, uteri removed from women undergoing hysterectomies are provided with oxygen and the necessary nutrients and hormones to mimic early pregnancy. They are used to "house" embryos, conceived through IVF, for the first few days of their development. A doctor in the U.S. recently received a patent for an "artificial uterus" designed to suspend a fetus in a liquid environment.[10]

More and more, the technologies already in place and those on the drawing board describe a future in which procreation would belong not to women but to a few highly specialized men who could, literally, control the means of production.

"Surplus" embryos, belonging to the (mostly) men who create them and determine their future, are a powerful symbol of how successful science has become in its attempts to control human procreation. As Varda Burstyn has written, "... the surplus embryo is not just a product of capitalist industrialization as it has engaged with procreation. It is also a product of masculinist science. It is the motherless embryo, the homonculus, the essence of human life that science has been seeking to find, to take over, to recreate. It is human life abstracted from mother and nature, now nurtured, sustained and soon to be shaped by doctors and technicians."[11]

When I began writing this piece, I spoke with my doctor to confirm the astonishing figures I had gotten from one text, on the numbers of eggs we possess. At first she doubted the numbers, convinced that they were too high. Then she pulled out a book she probably hadn't used since medical school and there were those same amazing numbers.

I've spoken to my doctor about the reproductive and genetic technologies many times in the last few years, and she has found lots of good articles for me from medical journals. She has her own strong feelings about these technologies.

They mostly come from her work in the sexually transmitted disease clinic that is part of a community health centre. Every day she treats young women suffering from chlamydia. The most insidious of the sexually transmitted diseases, chlamydia is often dangerously asymptomatic until it flares up as pelvic inflammatory disease, one of the major causes of infertility. (See also the article by Lynda Davies in Volume Two.)

A report released by The Advisory Committee on the Status of Women in 1990 predicts a 33 percent increase in infertility in the next group of young women coming into their childbearing years.[12] Sexually transmitted diseases are a major cause of the rise. This information doesn't surprise my doctor. She and her colleagues have been telling the government the same thing for years, but only after long battles did Quebec finally begin paying for chlamydia treatment in April 1992.

The Advisory Committee document also reported that in 1987 the federal government spent $3.5 million on the new reproductive technologies and $400,000 on public health research into reproductive disorders.[13] That came as no surprise to my doctor either. After all, teenagers have little political clout.

When I tell my doctor about new technologies like *in vitro* maturation she gets both astonished and angry. "Who are these people?" she asks me. "They are like Frankenstein!"

Frankenstein. His name comes up often when I talk to people about reproductive technology. It is not surprising. The idea of man-made man has always captivated the imagination in a unique fashion, a mixture of both fear and fascination. By introducing the figure of the scientist as an agent of creation into the public imagination, Mary Shelley cast a visionary glance into the future and in the process created a modern myth. This is a tale with all the metaphoric depth and resonance of the classic myths, except we know exactly how and where this story came into being. We know the author, all about her life and her thoughts as she wrote this extraordinary book.

I confess I had never read Mary Shelley's book and perhaps never would have if it weren't for a lecture I went to a few years ago. Monette Vacquin is a French psychoanalyst. That afternoon she swept us through a rapid description of Mary Shelley's life and her work, moved us on to an analysis of Nazi ideology, and then linked it all to the new reproductive technologies. Struggling back to earth after her lecture I was relieved to hear that the ground she covered that day was in her book, *Frankenstein ou les délires de la raison* (*Frankenstein or the nightmares of reason*),[14] and that I could travel the terrain again at my own speed.

But before I began, I read Mary Shelley's *Frankenstein*. I admit that I had grown up with the classic-comic, Hollywood version of the story, so reading the original was a revelation.

When a kid dresses up like Frankenstein for Halloween, he's not going to put on glasses and a white lab coat. He'll stick bolts on his forehead and shoulder pads under his sweat shirt. But Victor Frankenstein wasn't that kind of monster. And as for Mary's monster, the one with no name, well, he was a surprise. Not the demented, random killer we think of, but a creature overcome by the torment and despair of his loneliness. Driven by his suffering he becomes a murderer, but a very selective one, setting out to create a void, an emptiness around Frankenstein, the man who created him and then so heartlessly abandoned him.

In a bad week it feels like not a day has gone by without the papers reporting yet another experimental manipulation of the human psyche: creating children born to their grandmothers or to women old enough to be grandmothers, or babies conceived from the gametes of their siblings or carried by their sisters — all brought to us by doctors hiding behind a self-constructed rationale designed to turn experiment into medical treatment. This reckless toying with human nature has already been so banalized that it is not the topic of social criticism, but of movies and soap operas!

I think if we are to fully understand the dangers in these new reproductive experiments we need to consider them in light of all that makes us human. We cannot afford to ignore the realm of the imagination, or avoid the unquantifiable when we measure the impact of these technologies. After all, one of our most compelling fantasies, human creation without sex, without an intimate relationship with another person, has now moved irretrievably from the psychic to the physical world.

Vacquin's book is an excellent vehicle from which to begin that exploration. I've given up hope that it will ever be translated (which is certainly our loss), so I will humbly attempt to interpret some of her ideas.

What did Mary Shelley know, Vacquin asks? How is it that this young woman was able to look so clearly at her present and predict the future? Mary saw that the monstrousness lay not in the creature but in the creator, he who was able to give actual life to his desire, he who would shape human life to his own ends. She unmasked the obsession to control which lay behind the scientists' alibi of a thirst for knowledge. She saw the desire for power in the exercise of intelligence and in the corruption of its use. Mary's warning is not about the monsters we create but about the monsters we risk becoming when creation becomes a laboratory act, separated from sex and love, this essential human experience that is at once a physical encounter with another person and a loss of control. What had Victor Frankenstein lost that he was searching so hard to find? What led him to create this monster, a thing with no name, no mother or father, no childhood, no memory? An object on which Victor can turn all the curiosity which he is incapable of turning on himself, unable to ask himself who he is, and where he comes from? Why had he chosen a scalpel as the tool with which to search for his origins?

With his solitary deed, his removal of the relationship with a woman from the act of creation, Victor puts out into the world something which will destroy all possibility of relationships in his own life. Soon he is left with no father, no friends, no wife and no country. All that remains is Victor and his question, Victor and his answer. But unlike Victor, these modern day Frankensteins, the LIFE[15] doctors and GIFT[16] givers do not just change their own world. They are transforming ours, manipulating the most fundamental of all our human relationships.

Vacquin writes extensively about the "abolition of the metaphor" and its implications. Now that science can make real our most extreme dreams and fantasies, is there any place left for our imagination? And what have we lost when we lose that ground?

Taken in to watch an egg retrieval in an IVF clinic, Vacquin writes, "When the surgeon signals me to come forward, I see that I am placed at the head of the woman who is lying there, at just the right place to listen to her. But today she is sleeping silently. As a psychoanalyst, I am used to having bodies laid out in front of me, and in my office it is often also a question of what is going on in their belly. It sometimes even happens that what they say there will result in the birth of children. But what takes place in this operating room is in the 'literal sense' and I am familiar only with the 'figurative sense.' I shiver in spite of the heat in the operating room. This universe without metaphor is not mine."

Myths and fantasies are now medical/scientific realities. Women give birth to their son's children and are hailed as surrogate grandmothers. Here the myth of Frankenstein is replaced by that of Oedipus and Jocasta, except that story ended in ruin not celebration.

Considering the dismal success rates, Vacquin suggests that the real attraction of IVF is its imaginative content.

In the years since the birth of the first "test tube" baby, the entire catalogue of infantile fantasies, nightmares and myths about our origins have been given life through science:

* My parents aren't my parents.

* My mother is a virgin.

* My father is a powerful magician.

* You can buy babies from a store.

* I am not the results of anyone else's sexual act.

These fragmented forms of conception wipe out the differences between genders and even generations. But to become healthy independent individuals, children need to find their place in relation to these differences. If they have been removed by technology, or so confused as to make them impossible to locate, what opportunity does the child have to ever understand herself in relationship to others?

If we so profoundly transform the way we "do it" — the way we make babies — we cannot help but transform who we are, and what we will become. This is what Mary knew.

NOTES

This paper is based on a talk I gave at a workshop on Women and Technology at McMaster University, Hamilton, Ontario.

1   Gena Corea, "What the King cannot see," paper delivered to the Law Reform Commission of Victoria, May 1986.
2   *Ibid.*
3   Deborah Jones, "N.S. hospital set to try transplant of fetal tissue to treat Parkinson's," the *Globe and Mail*, February 15, 1990.
4   Stephen Strauss, "Fetal brain tissue to be grown in labs, U.S. scientists say," the *Globe and Mail*, February 15, 1990.
5   Andrew Kimbrell, *The Human Body Shop*, Harper, San Francisco, 1993.
6   Richard Saltus, "Korean doctors report in-vitro fertilization breakthrough," the *Boston Globe*, November 15, 1989.
7   *Ibid.*
8   *Ibid.*
9   Stephen Strauss, "Fetal brain tissue to be grown in labs, U.S. scientists say," the *Globe and Mail*, February 15, 1990.
10 Sabra Chartrand, "Patents. For premature babies born in the second trimester, hope of survival in an artificial uterus," the *New York Times*, July 19, 1993.
11 Varda Burstyn, "Making Babies," *Canadian Forum* Magazine, March 1992.
12 Heather Bryant, *The Infertility Dilemma. Reproductive Technologies and Prevention*. The Canadian Advisory Council on the Status of Women, Ottawa, 1990.
13 *Ibid.*
14 Monette Vacquin, *Frankenstein ou les délires de la raison*, Ed. François Bourin, Paris, 1989.
15 The LIFE (Laboratory Initiated Fetal Emplacement) Program is the name of the IVF clinic at the Toronto East General Hospital.
16 GIFT (gamete intrafallopian transfer, an assisted reproduction technique).

2

WORRYING — AND WORRYING ABOUT — THE GENETICIZATION OF REPRODUCTION AND HEALTH

Abby Lippman

Biomedical researchers are today redefining human geography. These modern explorers are elaborating a new map of humans, a map based on genes that is likely to alter our views of the world — and our place in it — even more profoundly than did the maps generated by Columbus and other 15th and 16th century explorers. This mapmaking has already begun to alter our perceptions of self and other, of normality and abnormality, and to change our concepts of cause and prevention. This is probably more so in the area of reproduction than any other. This paper stems from work in progress in which I am examining the stories being told by today's colonizers, scientists, about their explorations and about the new world of disease, health and reproduction they are defining.

Let me note right away that I use the word "stories" not to suggest that what scientists are saying is not true; this may or may not be the case. Rather, I use it in a literary not a legal sense to capture the idea that how scientists present their observations and study results is no different from how novelists present their interpretations of the external world. Both sets of storytellers tame, shape and interpret "raw" material to convey a message, with the constructions of each reflecting their prior beliefs and the prevailing social/cultural context. The stories told by scientists, therefore, are as appropriately objects of analysis as are the stories of other writers, and the stories in which I am especially interested deal with matters of health and disease.

Judging by headlines in newspapers and titles of articles in professional journals, today's stories on these issues are being told increasingly in the language of genetics. Using the metaphor of blueprints or texts, genes and DNA fragments are presented as a set of instructions to make us who and what we are, with zealots going so far as to describe human diseases as "typographical errors" (Shapiro, 1990). Through these stories, which are beginning to threaten seriously other narratives, geneticists and others are conditioning how we name, view and propose to manage a whole host of disorders and disabilities, with "genetics" increasingly identified as the way to reveal and explain health and disease, normality and abnormality (e.g. Baird, 1990). These stories are already directing how intellectual and financial resources are applied to resolve health problems but, even more critically, they are profoundly influencing our values and attitudes.

To capture this process, and to summarize the major theme of the stories, I have begun to use the term "geneticization." Very briefly, I define as geneticization the ongoing process that includes the ever-growing tendencies to name things that distinguish one person from another as genetic in origin, to reduce differences between individuals to their DNA codes and to define most disorders, behaviors and physiological variations as at least partly genetic in origin. It involves the use of genetic tools to look for differences between people and the application of genetic interventions and services to resolve multiple health and social problems.

Geneticization is social and political as well as — maybe even more than it is — biomedical. It is also a process of colonization insofar as genetic technologies and approaches are applied to areas not necessarily genetic. Its most costly expression is the international genome program to map and sequence the 50,000 - 100,000 human genes (see appendix); its most widespread application thus far is prenatal diagnosis which comprises the multiple screening and testing procedures used to assess the physical status of the fetus or embryo during — if not before — a woman's pregnancy.

Geneticization places more and more areas of women's experiences under the territorial control of genetics, subject to genetic ideas about both the conditions for and the quality of life. While geneticization does not reverberate identically for all women, some general issues do appear to cut across racial, income, social status, ethnic and ability differences and I emphasize these common matters when I suggest it is important for us to *"worry"* about the process and the technologies of genetic screening and testing it engenders. Moreover, it is important to worry in both the 20th and the 16th century senses of the word. We must not only reflect on certain "anxieties, troubles and uneasinesses" many have with geneticization and the activities it fosters, but must also "assault verbally" the discourse of geneticization and of genetic screening to challenge their meaning.

I will orient my worrying here primarily around some selected aspects of the genetic screening of fetuses (or embryos) that concern me and the women and genetic counselors interviewed in our ongoing studies. I will also worry (about), but more briefly, genetic testing of other kinds. But first let me say unequivocally that the targets of my critique are practices, not people; ideologies, not individuals. To the degree that separation is possible, my focus is on public policies, not private practices; on collective values, not individual ethics. I do not seek to find fault with those who use prenatal or other genetic services. In fact, I admire their courage in grappling concretely with issues I, fortunately, need mostly face academically.

PRENATAL TESTING

Before I consider some general sources to, and of, worry, some background about prenatal testing may be useful.

Examination of the fetus in utero probably first occurred almost 100 years ago when an x-ray picture was taken of a dead fetus. However, prenatal screening and diagnosis as we think of them now have been available "routinely" to certain groups of women, selectively to others, only since amniocentesis was first performed about twenty to twenty-five years ago.

Amniocentesis and the other technologies of prenatal screening and diagnosis currently in use provide access to fetal cells and amniotic fluid and enable the visualization of the developing fetus. Using these technologies, all recognizable chromosomal variations, many selected developmental malformations, over 150 biochemical disorders, and fetal sex can be detected before birth, with the list continuing to expand and the techniques being applied earlier and earlier in pregnancy. If prenatal diagnosis were first used for conditions generally regarded by physicians as "serious," and for which there were no effective treatments, as developers claim, it is now available for conditions with little or uncertain impact on postnatal health and functioning; for conditions that will appear, if at all, only in adulthood; and for conditions for which no treatment exists. The speed with which these new technologies have been adopted into clinical practice and the growing number of women to whom they are applied are staggering.

Amniocentesis is, to date, the most widely used procedure for obtaining fetal cells. Performed at about sixteen to twenty weeks' gestation, with studies underway to assess the safety of its earlier use, amniocentesis involves the insertion of a thin hollow needle through a woman's abdomen and into the amniotic sac to remove a small sample of fluid surrounding the developing fetus. This fluid contains cells from the fetus. Once stimulated to multiply in the laboratory, these cells can then be analyzed to determine the number of chromosomes they contain, the fetal sex, and the presence of DNA sequences associated with certain specific conditions. The growth and analysis of the fetal cells may take as long as three to four weeks so that women who decide to terminate their pregnancies following test results do not obtain an abortion until about the twentieth week, which is halfway through the pregnancy.

Chorionic villus sampling (CVS) is another way of obtaining fetal cells for diagnosis. It was said to be developed specifically to permit prenatal testing earlier in pregnancy. In CVS, a small tube (catheter) is inserted through a woman's vagina and cervix. It is then advanced under ultrasound guidance until it reaches the placenta from which a small amount of tissue (chorionic villi) is removed. Any chromosomal or DNA change can, in theory, be diagnosed with tissues obtained by CVS because the cells of the fetus and the placenta (which are formed from chorionic villi) are genetically the same.

CVS can be done as early as ten weeks after a woman's last menstrual period and, while the results of tests carried out on placental tissue could be available within hours, at least a two or three day waiting period — and more often longer — is usually required. Even so, if a woman decides to end her pregnancy following CVS, the abortion can be carried out in the first trimester. The "price" of this earlier intervention includes the somewhat less accurate test results with cells obtained from CVS than from amniocentesis, the more frequent need to repeat the diagnostic procedure following CVS, the likelihood that many women who would otherwise have a spontaneous abortion (miscarriage) must now themselves make painful decisions about continuing or terminating their pregnancies and persisting uncertainty about its total safety.

In Canada, where they are covered by public funds, the use of amniocentesis and CVS have been generally restricted to women whose age (usually 35 years, a completely arbitrary criterion) is said to put them at increased risk for having a child with Down syndrome — a group that comprises about 80-90 percent of all women currently tested — and for women known to be at risk of having a child with some specific condition that can be diagnosed via fetal cells or amniotic fluid. Neither of these two tests is done "routinely" in other groups of women.

By contrast, almost all women experience another form of prenatal testing (even if it is not so-labeled) if they have access to and receive what has become part of a standard package of prenatal care: *ultrasound examinations* (see Mitchell, this book). During these exams, now carried out earlier and earlier in pregnancy, high frequency sound waves are projected into the uterus and the sound waves that are reflected back are resolved visually to allow one to "see" the fetus on a television-like screen (and the photograph of this image often offered to a woman as the first entry for her "baby book" is now supplemented by the sale of a videotape of the "real time" scan). As a tool for prenatal diagnosis, ultrasound can be used to identify certain malformations in fetuses known to be at risk for one of these abnormalities. It can also be used to identify fetal sex. Most subtle malformations will not be identified when ultrasound is applied on a non-diagnostic basis for pregnancy dating although more obvious changes in the body shape and size of the fetus should be detectable.

Apparently on its way to becoming another universal technology for prenatal screening in Canada, is the withdrawal of a sample of blood from a pregnant woman and its analysis for the presence of alpha-fetoprotein (AFP) and, in some jurisdictions, a limited number of other serum constituents that tend to be found in increased or decreased levels when the fetus has, respectively, a malformation of the neural tube or Down syndrome. This *MS-AFP (maternal serum AFP)* analysis, performed about 16 weeks from the first day of a woman's last menstrual period before becoming pregnant, is not diagnostic. It has rather poor predictive value and, at most, only identifies women at slightly higher than average risk of having a child with one of these conditions. Most women whose initial screening results are considered to be abnormal do not have fetuses with the conditions sought, but this is only learned after the completion of confirmatory tests (ultrasound and amniocentesis) which are recommended to all in this group to establish the diagnosis (and after these women have experienced at least a fair amount of anxiety in the interim). The application of MS-AFP screening irrespective of a woman's prior risk of having a fetus with a neural tube defect or Down syndrome in community-wide programs is acknowledged to be the first mass prenatal genetic screening (which the routine ultrasound scanning of all pregnant women is not) and is already underway in several parts of Canada.

Beyond these "established" technologies are others under development and already beginning to be marketed. A growing number of investigators have begun to report their ability to obtain and make diagnoses from *fetal cells in the mother's circulation.* With the use of increasingly sophisticated technologies, these cells, which have crossed the placental barrier and entered a woman's bloodstream, can be separated from the woman's blood cells, grown in the laboratory, subjected to procedures that amplify their genetic material, and stained with specific (fluorescent) dyes to locate the presence or absence of DNA sequences. This appears to be an "up-and-coming" approach for prenatal diagnosis, and if it does provide accurate results, it would, in principle, allow what is now a "routine" for pregnant women — having a blood sample taken — to replace a medically sophisticated and much more invasive procedure such as amniocentesis or CVS for obtaining fetal cells for prenatal diagnosis.

Another approach that may proliferate in the future is *embryo or pre-implantation diagnosis.* In this approach, which is already used in programs of technological reproduction in conjunction with IVF (and for animals as well as women; see the chapter by Basen in the section about eugenics), a very early embryo is removed from a pregnant woman (or first created in the laboratory following *in vitro* fertilization), tested, and, if it "passes," (re)placed in the uterus to continue its development. This technology has so far only been used in Canada as a research tool for the diagnosis of certain specific genetic disorders in embryos but, should it appear not to harm the child-to-be, its further application has been endorsed by many researchers. And, given that its advocates have domesticated this problematic technique by affixing it with the acronym "BABI" (blastocyst analysis before implantation) and then declaring it to be, potentially, a particularly welcome approach because it will circumvent abortion — only "unaffected" embryos would be (re)implanted — broader application is not an unrealistic expectation. After all, those developing prenatal testing techniques have consistently assumed, despite the absence of data on the subject, that "earlier is better." In other words, that it is "better" to know before than at or after birth that something is "wrong" with the fetus; even "better" to obtain this information earlier rather than later in pregnancy; and still "better" to know the status of the fetus before a pregnancy begins because by transferring only "good" embryos the need for abortion (of "bad" embryos??) can be averted.

Unfortunately, this technology cannot be considered in any depth here, but I think it essential to worry (about) pre-implantation diagnosis. It represents a marriage between reproductive and genetic technologies and a potential offspring of this union is germline gene manipulation. For, once the fertilized egg is outside a woman's body, it is accessible to those wanting to experiment with it, and an increasingly popular area for experimentation today involves the introduction of genetic material into human cells.

WHAT'S THE WORRY

Given the collection of techniques available — and only those most likely to be used in other than rare situations have been described — there seems good reason to worry (about) geneticization, and one way to begin is to consider what these technologies mean to and for women and their childbearing.

Most generally, they raise a number of fundamental concerns related to women's health and health care simply because how, when, why, to and by whom they are applied will be conditioned by prevailing attitudes about women, their bodies and their social roles. So long as procreation, pregnancy and motherhood are (still) seen as central to being a woman in our sexist society, women will experience testing not merely as parents, but in ways peculiar to being *mothers* of children, ways that usually cut across traditional distinctions between us. And, because the world in which genetic and other reproductive technologies are developing is gendered, these technologies cannot be neutral or escape gendered use.

Thus, I worry from the start about how societal powers and privileges embedded in local screening practices shape women's plans for and experiences of maternity. Women are already, if differentially, disadvantaged, generally powerless, vulnerable to offers of services because of their diminished status, challenged by prejudicial norms surrounding motherhood and delegated responsibility for family health, and prenatal diagnosis cannot but be influenced by — and itself influence — these features of our lives. Furthermore, women have not played a major role in developing these techniques, but as children's primary caregivers, may become beholden to their use.

Beyond this, I worry because already, prenatal testing has been naturalized through stories which describe it as only a response to pregnant women at "genetic risk" who "need" some reassurance, as something women "choose" (see Lippman, 1986). But these reports, as all "stories" about prenatal testing, are not records of experiences so much as they are ways to produce meanings and so I worry about the use of these words in this context.

In North America today, where major responsibility for family health care is still allocated to women who alone are expected to do all that is recommended or available for the sake of their children, it is not surprising that a woman offered ultrasound or serum screening by an expert who implies that she really wants to have a healthy child (doesn't she?) perceives a *need* to be tested, to do all that is recommended. But can we really know if her agreement to testing in such a context is an expression of choice, an instance of conformity or a response to coercion?

Certainly, reports about prenatal testing hide the second and third possibilities (conformity and coercion) when considerations of the (macro and micro) constraints and expectations in which needs arise and choice occurs are absent from them. How and by whom has need been constructed, has choice been defined?

The interpretation of "need" is always political. Thus, feminists and others who question the prevailing interpretations and the extent of choice provided by the current practice of prenatal testing are seeking *not* to limit women's options, but to enlarge their number, insure their availability and involve women in their creation. To these critics, myself included, choice in prenatal testing requires not merely that women can themselves opt for a particular procedure but that women who reject the process are not questioned about their motives more than are women who agree immediately to testing, which is not how the women we have interviewed describe their experiences. It means that a woman can continue her pregnancy after a fetal diagnosis is made because help to support a child with a disability is guaranteed, which is not what the women we talk to perceive. And, it means that personal actions are completely severed from public agendas so that a *decrease* in "uptake" rates of testing from current levels might be seen to measure the success, not the failure, of prenatal screening, which is not how geneticists now view usage (cf Clarke, 1990).

In fact, in exploring the matter of choice in prenatal testing even further, it may be that the process in North America actually impedes or restricts free decision-making and choice. Let me explain.

In general, our reviews of medical genetics texts and of material presented to women considering the possibility of prenatal testing show that these documents convey only partial information in their highly charged stories about Down syndrome (Lippman and Brunger, 1992); about the disease-preventing capabilities of fetal diagnosis; and about the routine nature of this intervention. By aiming at entirely legitimate desires (of all women for a healthy child) and normative (if not self-serving) beliefs (that medical technology provides a way to fulfil these desires), offers of prenatal testing leave little opportunity for a woman to reflect meaningfully and develop her own knowledge of and opinions about Down syndrome or testing. Even when genetic counseling is provided prior to prenatal diagnosis (and with the huge expansion in testing programs this is becoming less and less common), the discussion is directed towards the technology, not to the range of possibilities for the pregnant woman 35 years of age or older. "Counseling," when it is provided at all, is programed into the use of the technology rather than made available independently of this agenda. How else to explain the situation where only the women who *decline* screening are referred for genetic counseling in some jurisdictions (Green et al., 1993), where only the women who *reject* parts of the antenatal care package — if they are white and well-educated — are treated as somehow "abnormal." It would appear as if medical care providers take a Caucasian, middle-class, biomedical perspective as the norm and more easily allow African-Canadian and Asian-Canadian women to opt out, apparently assuming that *their* rejection of testing must reflect some ethnic difference from "us" to which we should be sensitive.

The minimal concern with informed choice in prenatal testing seems reflected, too, in how both the women and the counselors we have interviewed seem to regard their concerns about and reluctance towards testing as obstacles to decision-making rather than as valid expressions of the moral malaise the procedures arouse. And, it is reflected further in our observation that genetic counselors take a positive response to their question, "Have you ever heard of Down syndrome?" as sufficient evidence that a woman planning to be tested is informed about the reasons for testing. (For more on this, see the chapter by Goundry.)

Most counseling is provided by a genetics counselor in a genetics clinic[1] (cf Scutt, 1991), and usually with enormous time pressures because of limits on what stage of pregnancy in which testing can be carried out, a situation and set of circumstances that do not foster reasoned reflection. (A not dissimilar situation exists when women who have failed to conceive as quickly as they had hoped receive counseling only in an infertility clinic; when contraceptive advice is given in a population control rather than a family planning program.)

Thus, while a woman may only exceptionally be told directly to be tested or to abort, and consequently most can give the appearance of choosing, any empowerment these women have is primarily provisional and conditional. In a society where warning labels and public advertisements constantly remind women that what they do can harm the fetus, but that if they behave responsibly, they can reduce this harm, offers of prenatal screening and testing are hardly "neutral" and even, perhaps, impossible to refuse (except for a very determined few). There are rewards and sanctions, both implicit and explicit, that invite and encourage their use. (This theme is developed further in the chapter by Maria Barile.)

MORE TO WORRY (ABOUT)

Prenatal testing programs express the historically-based nexus between control over reproduction and control over heredity — with the nexus located in women's bodies. Whatever may be claimed as motives, therefore, prenatal testing cannot but be eugenic. These programs are for detecting and preventing the birth of certain babies, in fact for "gatekeeping." This is most evident when the diagnosis of embryos obtained following *in vitro* fertilization and the transfer of only the "good ones" is proposed as an "advance" in prenatal testing. Even if proponents of this supposed "advance" did not generally ignore the physical risks to a woman and the documented poor success of IVF interventions in advocating it, their single-minded attention to the embryo, to what is really a quality-controlled embryo, clearly links reproductive with genetic control. (Gwynne Basen shows this in her chapter in the eugenics section.)

But the linkage exists, too, though perhaps more subtly, in claims that routine prenatal testing is reassuring. This claim may be statistically justified, since the vast majority of fetuses will not have what is being sought, but beyond ignoring the high frequencies of false positive test results when prenatal screening is carried out in the general population of pregnant women and the anxiety these generate, it nevertheless assumes abortion when a fetus does have the condition sought; spending most of one's pregnancy awaiting the birth of a child with a detected variation does not really seem likely to allay a woman's concerns.

Related to this, and another aspect of prenatal testing to worry, and worry about, is the way stories about it restrict disability to being simply a medical problem. Much research shows that disability, most of which is not of prenatal onset, only becomes of major consequence when prevailing social, economic and political policies do not allow for a wide range of abilities and convert impairments into handicaps. Prenatal testing implicitly assumes some norm of ability, hides the social roots and political practices that create handicap and reshapes the problem of disability so that it need not be *ours* collectively to solve — what will *we* do to embrace and accommodate those among us who have or will develop disabilities? — but becomes one for an individual woman to prevent — what will *she* do to avoid having a baby who has or will develop a disability? The individual is made into an agent of the state, and this is explicit (as is the fragility of our claims of neutrality) when a 38-year-old woman gives birth to a baby with Down syndrome and we ask — even if only among ourselves, as Elizabeth Thompson has noted — why she didn't get tested.

In addition, by orienting prenatal screening specifically to the detection of particular conditions, we explicitly make a social statement about the quality or the value of a fetus and on the adult it may grow up to be based solely on its genetic/chromosomal material. Our programs say it is okay if children with certain chromosomes are not born, that being at risk to develop a particular condition is, in effect, worse than being alive (Asch, 1988). And we restate this view when we count the abortion of a fetus with some disorder as a core benefit, not a worrisome cost, in our conventional economic analyses of screening programs (cf. Modell and Kuliev, 1991).

Further, and despite our rhetoric of choice, the power to set boundaries, to make value judgments about who may or may not be born, remains disproportionately with the university researchers and for-profit laboratories developing and deploying the technologies of testing. Only the conditions for which they make tests available can be sought — with what is available determined, as in all colonialism, by prevailing social values as well as by personal goals for professional recognition or financial profit.

Medical care providers further influence attitudes to what health and abnormality mean and who should be born by what they tell parents about genetic conditions — and these tellings appear to come in what Ben Wilfond and I have called "twice-told" ways (Lippman and Wilfond, 1992). For example, the information provided to those who are considering genetic testing for Down syndrome and for cystic fibrosis differs strikingly from that provided to those who have given birth to a child with one of the conditions. In both circumstances, the overall information is correct. However, the *before* testing information is largely negative, oriented to avoiding the birth of a child with Down syndrome or cystic fibrosis by focusing on technical matters and the array of potential medical complications and physical limitations that may occur in children with the condition, while the *after* birth information tends to be more positive, oriented to caring for a child with one of these conditions by focusing on compensating aspects of the condition, highlighting the availability of medical and social resources and stressing hope for the future.

We worry about separate before and after stories and what this may signify. Granted, no single story, however balanced, can ever be neutral or value-free. But why have we chosen to tell different stories? Why not just one?

The different versions of these stories remind us that even if individual women can choose to be tested or to abort, their options have first been created by the deeds and words of others. That the birth of certain babies should be avoided would appear to be embedded inextricably in geneticists' messages no less than in the medium of testing. This should worry us enough, I suggest, that we continually question our own values and consider why aborting a fetus on the basis of its ability — its particular value[2] — is not only socially acceptable but actually encouraged. Why have we made Down syndrome, for example, a privileged reason for prenatal screening and abortion? What else shall we so privilege? If raising children with disabilities is the problem, is prenatal screening the answer? Why have we converted a problem in society — inability to accommodate disability — into a problem in the fetus?

Legitimate efforts to help a woman have a healthy baby are essential. But if healthy children really matter to us, as we say they do, does prenatal testing represent our best effort? At the collective level, the birth prevalence of low birth weight is far greater than the birth prevalence of Down syndrome or neural tube defects. Why have efforts to find every fetus with Down syndrome become so important to us that universal triple screening is entering recommended medical practice,[3] while ensuring early prenatal care for all women is still an unachieved goal? Why has preventing neural tube defects become so important that universal folate supplementation is proposed, while sufficient income and nutrition to all (pregnant) women to decrease their probability of having a baby with growth retardation is still not guaranteed? The well-being of children is inseparable from the well-being of women, and social, political and economic neglect of women interferes more with the physical and mental development of their children than the genes they inherit.

If healthy children really do matter, we must end this neglect and create the conditions in which women's agency and their choices can be fully exercised.

Thus, we should worry about prenatal testing when relying on it to insure our children's health at the collective level threatens to displace attention from society's role in creating illness. If we worry, even a bit, perhaps we will delay our initial excitement about the potential to obtain and make diagnoses from single fetal cells in maternal blood samples until the presuppositions underlying suggestions to expand prenatal screening with this approach have been uncovered, until the ways in which such screening will be of consequence to pregnant women have been explored and until the place for this screening among our overall health priorities has been debated.

POSTNATAL GENETIC TESTING: ANOTHER WORRY

The ways in which practitioners construct individuals as patients with (or at risk of having) some disorder and who and what they label (as ill or abnormal) is necessarily contingent on time and place, and the "place" for today's labelling is increasingly the genetic map being drawn in a society that remains deeply fractured along lines of gender, race, class and ability. Whereas "energetic physicians" once "discerned microorganisms responsible for almost every ill known to mankind[sic]" (Rosenberg, 1992), their latter day heirs discern genes. I worry about giving genes prominence in contemporary constructions of health and disorder because social, political and ethical claims will be quite different when a condition is seen as a failure of our genes rather than as a failure, for example, in providing essential resources for health.

I worry, too, because despite the biological reality of human disease and the serious need for efforts to reduce the suffering and costs associated with it, biological processes, disorders and disabilities are not merely physiological or physical states with fixed contours. They are social products with variant shapes and distributions that are fashioned, interpreted and given meaning according to beliefs, attitudes, values and interests. There is no strictly objective and value-free view of the biological world of health and disease. All explanations of it are shaped by the historical and cultural setting within which they are offered. Furthermore, the same observations may be taken as evidence to construct very different images of disease and ill health, very different etiological hypotheses or stories, with that which is chosen reflecting — and imbued with — the assumptions, vested interests and ideology of the investigators and those funding them (e.g. Tesh, 1988; Payer, 1989).[4]

What, then, may be the effects of emphasizing genetics as the basis of human variation, of choosing genetics for the representation of health problems and testing individuals for genes that may make them more likely than someone else to develop some disorder? Should we worry (about) them?

Without question, the map of the human genome currently being drafted will identify variations in DNA patterns. Genes said to "cause" disease as well as those associated with increased susceptibility to specific disorders, will be claimed to have been found. But identification of the exact chromosomal location of a segment of DNA, even complete knowledge of the base sequences it comprises, will allow only the determination of its presence in a specific person. It does not — and cannot — foretell what that person will be like. Human individuality is more than personal biology. And genes do not "cause" anything although they do make some things possible. So, even if the DNA pattern is clearly associated with some disease or disorder, knowing where it is will neither predict the severity of the condition nor solve the health problem(s) that affect those with the gene.

The widely used example of sickle cell anemia illustrates clearly the limits of isolated genetic information. The exact DNA alteration associated with this condition was identified over 20 years ago. Nevertheless, predicting beforehand the extent or frequency of crises or quality of life of any particular person is still impossible — and a cure remains elusive. If this is the situation for sickle cell anemia, a so-called "simple" disorder, there is little reason to expect mapping will be any more "useful" for far more prevalent and complex physical and mental conditions now being brought (inappropriately, if colonially) under a genetic rubric (e.g. high blood pressure, alcoholism, Alzheimer disease, breast cancer). A gene or genes associated with these variations may be found. (Many are certainly actively searching for them.) But, what then? Will we necessarily know more that is pertinent to a person's health with respect to these conditions when these genes are mapped than we would without this specific information? Will we want to know via prenatal diagnosis who has these genes?

At most, traits may be influenced by genes; trite, but still true, biology is not destiny. Thus, no matter how refined, even a complete "genetic profile" of an individual is not a blueprint and will reveal very little about how the person will turn out. Consequently, claims for the urgency of mapping for individual health may contain more hyperbole than reality about what is needed to reduce illness.

Furthermore, by emphasizing the advantages, even the necessity, of creating an individualized genetic profile for each of us, the messages of geneticization direct the search for solutions to health problems in troubling ways. Simply by their enormous costs, gene mapping programs will absorb funds and energies that might have been applied to developing other possible stories about and interventions relevant to health and illness. In addition, by making it seem that there is no other approach and that our most pressing health problems, if not all of them — as well as a whole range of human variability — are "genetic," these messages erase the extent to which most socially important health conditions and behaviors are not determined by genetic factors alone. They make us forget the many factors that influence health — e.g. our social and physical environments, economic conditions, available health services — and that these, and not just genes, could be the subject of a program to reduce human suffering. And this is equally so for those with a genetic "predisposition" to develop some disorder. They, too, must experience some event or exposure (usually of unknown nature at present) for their gene(s) to be expressed.

Consequently, it is not immediately apparent that we need to know where genes are located to improve the overall health of a population or to promote the well-being of individuals, to understand illness, or to relieve suffering. We could, in fact, "map" the environment for sources of "susceptibility" instead of mapping the genome.

But this approach is forgotten in the attractively-phrased, medically-oriented arguments advanced by biomedical researchers to legitimize their genetic activities. They increasingly justify gene mapping by emphasizing the application of genetic information for the prediction and prevention of health problems, and we should worry about this. Does this justification not itself incorporate some troubling conceptual and social consequences (beyond the obviously and overtly eugenic ones)?

Construction of a human gene map will foster the identification of ever more variations between people, variations that can be sought in pre- and postnatal genetic screening programs. Among these variations will be DNA sequences that appear to be associated with a person's probability of developing some disorder at an unknown time in the future.

At first glance, mapping genes for susceptibility to complex and frequent conditions and implementing screening programs to identify those with these genes might appear to make sense. After all, individuals could then be informed about their probability of developing the disease in question and counseled about (behavioural) changes they should make to reduce their chance of becoming sick. For instance, if genetic testing were to identify a person thought to have an above average risk of developing high blood pressure, this individual could be advised to take measures with respect to her diet, leisure activities and occupational tasks that were thought to lower this probability and thus she might be able to avert that for which she is allegedly at increased risk.

On the basis of such arguments, claims are now made that early identification and early intervention will be "preventive." But, does the preference given to genetic screening as preventive medicine survive scrutiny? Does screening for genetic susceptibility really "make sense," and to whom? Does the identification of genetic — rather than other — difference(s) for susceptibility better serve those who get grouped and ranked qualitatively, with not all characteristics and endowments considered of equal value, or those in power, since they control the markers chosen, the populations to be investigated and the values assigned?

Examined closely, susceptibility screening that appears to make "sense" may merely make "cents" for those marketing testing kits while it strengthens inequities in health for the rest of us. Making "patients" of those who are well will generate extensive profits for biotech and pharmaceutical companies that first produce the tests we will all (be invited to) undergo and then develop "remedies" for the variations found, variations that will have suddenly become abnormalities — and the number of yet-to-be uncovered "vulnerabilities" we carry in our genes means that each of us will be "at risk" for something. And though enrolling individuals whose genes are said to put them "at risk" in education programs that emphasize the practice of "good lifestyle" behaviors to lower these risks may appear relevant and efficient, with this strategy already widely promoted in the literature, the reality is far more complex.

The social and political meaning of genetic testing, as well as its personal meaning, vary with the social/political position of the person to whom the technology is applied. Testing is integrated into health care and personal identity differentially according to the social status, economic power and political clout of the individual. For example, neither the ability (nor the desire) to change behaviour is distributed equally among all individuals. For those whose situation either embraces norms that differ from those of the white, middle class that currently prevail or who are unable to follow such rules it may not make "sense" to stop smoking, to relax, to exercise more and to follow a prudent diet, even after being identified as genetically at risk for a problem (such as heart disease) linked epidemiologically to these factors. Society does not permit all people, and especially not (all) women, to have the range of "lifestyle" choices the privileged have (even assuming we could agree on a definition of the term, "lifestyle"). Consider, for example, a single mother working rotating shifts in a chronic care hospital. She may be told to avoid stress and she may certainly want to. But is doing so a choice she can personally make? Can she control the timing and frequency of her children's illnesses and their conflict with her work schedule, a major source of recurrent stress as she tries to balance her multiple roles alone? The relationship between knowledge (including awareness of risk) and a decision to do something "healthy" is far more problematic than the reigning ideology would have us believe. And, the development and introduction of genetic technologies in an already stratified world means that they cannot escape stratified use.[5]

Thus, even if screening programs were known to work, and we lack published data that support such claims, in the context of the existing inequities in health which derive from class, gender, race and other social stratifications existing in Canada (and which themselves put people at risk for health problems), they are most likely to strengthen these stratifications. Again, not only will money be diverted from projects to correct these injustices, but emphasizing individual responsibility and change will likely erode the enthusiasm and support needed for developing social programs to reduce the risks to health clearly deriving from sexism, poverty and racism. The individual, not society, is seen to require change. A worrisome example of this occurs in a recent article in a medical journal describing the identification of a gene associated with susceptibility to lead poisoning and implying that this might be an appropriate target for a genetic screening program. Do we really need to find newborns (or fetuses) with this susceptibility? Lead poisoning is a major health problem, especially in the United States, and all efforts to prevent it should be given priority. However, is not the simplest, and least expensive solution, merely to replace the substandard housing, where lead-based paint is found, with decent accommodations?

Disease is not just the result of individual failure to follow advice. People do not choose to become ill. Babies who are well fed and have adequate housing do not eat the paint chipped off crumbling walls. Sensitive and accessible childcare policies ease some of the stress on working women. Existing cultural, political and economic restraints on options for dealing with matters of health and illness mean that obtaining and using information about one's genetic make-up and the ability to adopt any recommended practice will vary disproportionately in the population reflecting current inequities.[6] Society's choices may increase the likelihood of disease even more than individual choices.

This explains why gene mapping and molecular medicine, which seem so modern, may not necessarily open new ways to improve health but may merely revive a dated conception of preventive medicine by packaging it with an up-to-date image of prediction.

Further, to the degree that predictive medicine replaces society's responsibility to eliminate the adverse social circumstances damaging to health with the "susceptible" person's responsibility to avert that for which she is said to be at risk, to prevent a problem, it may be not just conservative but mischievous — if not harmful. The "predictive" model transfers accountability for health to the individual. It makes illness private and sets the stage for social control and for "victim blaming" of those who do not follow what is supposedly "sensible" advice for their health. Moreover, there may be no way to evaluate how "sensible" the advice actually is because barring massive randomized clinical trials, we will be unable to determine if those who followed recommendations and did not become ill stayed healthy because they behaved well or because their genes weren't really so "risky" after all.

CONCLUSION

Mapmaking, whether of the body or the earth, by scientists as by Columbus, is as much political and cultural as it is "scientific." The geneticization inscribed in the proliferating use of genetic and reproductive technologies contains certain inherent expectations about how, when and why these activities will be applied. Today's genome projects could not be done without the sophisticated technical machinery now available for studying DNA, but they would not be done if the reigning biomedical culture were not supportive of the genetic colonization — geneticization — currently in full force in the areas of health and illness. Carrying out these projects permits mapmakers, their funders and the purveyors of their products, today's "Isabellas and Ferdinands," to accrue tremendous power for defining how we think of ourselves and others, of health and disease, of normality and abnormality.

Justifying mapping as the way to improve health is doubtless an effective marketing strategy for molecular geneticists, pharmaceutical companies, manufacturers of laboratory equipment, insurance companies, police forces and genetic engineers, among others, but it closes the debate, suggesting we need only regulate the "costs" — broadly defined, it is true — to obtain all the benefits. But more than costs and benefits (economic and otherwise) are involved in assessing gene mapping. It may be ethical, but still dangerous. The genetic perspective itself, and not just its consequences, is problematic. As I have emphasized, it focuses attention on only certain selected features of individuals and makes only certain ways of dealing with their health-related problems seem appropriate. At a minimum, applying the genetic label to health problems automatically erases environmental and social factors that transform disease to illness, disability to handicap. The attention given to genome projects implies that biological factors are more important than social (or any other factor[s]) in disrupting health, and supporters of these projects fail to acknowledge that all ideas of causality are solidly linked to the prevailing economic and political beliefs and selected through a "grid of value judgments." They also do not question to whose advantage the genetic construction may be. Further, these projects necessarily entail a commitment to develop and apply biomedical technology for the solution of health problems, again foreclosing other ways to construct a response. Nowhere is this more obvious than in the proliferation of programs of prenatal and postnatal testing.

Some see geneticization producing only cures, prevention and benefits for patients. However, there are significant costs for those with health problems, too, when the narrow definitions of disease and restricted approaches to healing implicit in geneticization are applied. External control over procreation choices because of supposed risks to future generations, rejection from various job categories or inability to obtain health or life insurance because of one's genes are outcomes of geneticization that may not be as eagerly awaited as cures for disease, but *they* are not hypothetical.

In this context, defining a place for prenatal testing (as for postnatal screening and other genetic technologies) in our lives and in our health systems is not easy, perhaps because we've not yet asked enough fundamental questions. Our knowledge has not kept pace with our information. In the generation since the first in utero diagnosis of Down syndrome, we have accumulated a wealth of cytogenetic, biochemical and epidemiologic data about testing, but we still lack a common definition of the problems for which prenatal screening is said to be the solution and still do not know the full impact of prenatal testing on women's total health, power and social standing. Is it liberating or oppressive, or both?

It is naive to believe we can — or even would want to — unbite the apple or disinvent the technologies (though we might want to isolate rather than institutionalize them), but it is critical really to worry (new and old meanings) about them more. For example, we need to expose and explore the economic and eugenic forces propelling testing activities. Why do we increasingly describe genetic services as a public health matter and then give them high priority, when variations in the distribution of wealth and power have far greater impact on the distribution of health than do variations in the distribution of genes? Why do we rely on medical options for dealing with disorders, genetic or otherwise, rather than favour social policies or political practices required for health? Is "nature" really easier to change than "nurture" as geneticization implies?

Prenatal genetic testing, as other medical technologies, is especially seductive with its stories of human triumph. But triumphs for an individual are, unfortunately, not necessarily triumphs for the collectives to which she and we all belong. We must never lose our compassion for an individual's situation, but we must also not forget that addressing elastic private needs, needs that geneticists help to create, may distort our perspective and dislocate provisions required for our collective health or solidify existing inequities in women's positions. Individual rights may actually only have meaning within our relationships and collectivities.

Prenatal testing has a valence that varies with time and place. It is developed and applied with inherent expectations of how, when and why it will be used that are tied to attitudes about women and about disability. We need to question this technology — to worry it and to worry about it — because use and misuse here are not separable; and means and ends are in a circular relationship. As Nancy Press's data show so eloquently (Press and Browner, 1993), we have been complacent and have avoided discussing valence issues by framing screening as an approved medical matter even though (perhaps, because?) its controversial moral and social meanings are so troubling. This collective aphasia, too, is surely grounds for worry.

But we must do more than worry. We need rigorous public discussions to learn whether expansions of prenatal testing address problems that would better be solved otherwise than by transforming them into genetic problems. We need to consider if the allocation of resources to genetic services will correct gendered inequities and injustices in the health-care system that endanger women's and children's health and preferentially empower others. And we need to establish guarantees for the survival of diversity and progressive social development in this time of geneticization.

Women's desire for children without disability warrants our public and private support. However, this support must not itself do harm. Rather, it must truly enhance health. It must not measure its effectiveness by the short-term fix of money saved when the lives of those with present or future disabilities are prevented; it must nourish the diverse rather than eliminate the different; it must not view the birth of a child with a disability as a technological failure; and it must lead to a society that is not itself disabled or disabling. Does prenatal screening meet these criteria? Does geneticization provide this support?

In conclusion, let me repeat my belief that geneticization is as much political as biomedical; it is about economics as much as it is about basic science and it embraces eugenics as much, if not more than, it endorses treatment. Geneticization is fundamentally an institutionalized process for interpreting observations about health and illness and for distinguishing between me and you, us and the "other." Geneticization allows us to look for things of consequence in ways that create whole new groups of disorders, whole new groups of sufferers. But choosing the genetic direction today is as much in response to forces in society as to developments in science. Do we really want to go in this direction?

Merely by presenting genes on maps we set up barriers and restrictions. The gene maps will give us information about ourselves, but is it really very interesting information or more precisely, to whom will it be interesting? Instead of expanding our thoughts about illness and health, gene maps set up mental blinders and barriers, foster reductionism and establish a new basis for social control of individuals. More specifically, the map approach may be especially antithetical and unacceptable to women. Women have historically been "mapped" — i.e. defined and delineated by others, by men, with the assumption that once described they (we) will be knowable, predictable, manageable. Attempts to map women's "nature" have inevitably placed limits on what women can and should do. Do we want to extend these limits to all we can map?

Geneticization is mostly about the genes we transmit to our children. But our legacy to future generations is more than genetic. We also transmit certain values and beliefs, and these will influence the possibilities for our children and grandchildren no less than the genes they inherit.

Geneticization articulates certain values and perspectives. Developing in a society that is gendered, racist, classist and systematically discriminates against those with disabilities, it would be naive to think that how and for whom it is promoted and applied will not reflect and, in turn, reinforce these attitudes. Thus, geneticization necessarily influences how we think about and experience ourselves, our children and others, how we devise plans for healing and curing, how we define and deal with that we call "different," how we interrelate with our surrounding worlds. We might consider, therefore, what attitudes we want to perpetuate for ourselves or pass to our offspring.

Maps are a way to conquer nature. We are the nature geneticization seeks to conquer and so we need truly to ask what the process does to us — to how we think, how we interact, how we situate ourselves in the world. Do we want to conquer nature, to conquer ourselves? Or might we want to learn how we can best live with nature, with ourselves, infirmities and all? And, what stories do we want our children to tell our grandchildren?

APPENDIX: MAPPING AND SEQUENCING THE HUMAN GENOME

Directed research projects are underway worldwide to map and sequence the human genome. The genome represents all the genetic material in the chromosomes of an organism and the goal of mapping is to locate the 50,000 to 100,000 human genes (the exact number is not known for certain) on the 23 pairs of chromosomes. So far, about 2000 genes have been mapped. With changing techniques increasing the mapping rate (currently over 12 additional genes are located per week), a human gene map may be completed as predicted by the year 2005.

Sequencing, a distinct but interrelated activity, aims to identify the specific order of the approximately 3 billion pairs of nucleotide bases that make up the DNA molecules encoding the genetic material passed from parent to offspring. Its end product, a complete computerized "catalogue" of the genetic material of humans, will take longer to achieve.

SELECTED BIBLIOGRAPHY

Additional references can be found in my earlier publications; only a minority of those cited elsewhere have been included here.

Asch A (1988): "Reproductive technology and disability," in Cohen S, Taub N (eds): *Reproductive Laws for the 1990s*. Clifton, NJ: Humana Press, pp 59-101.

Baird P (1990): "Genetics and health care: A paradigm shift." *Perspect Biol Med* 33:203.

Clarke A (1990): "Genetics, ethics and audit". *Lancet* 335:1145-1147.

Green J, Snowdon C, Statham H (1993): "Pregnant women's attitudes to abortion and pre-natal screening." *J Reprod & Infant Psychol*, in press.

Lippman A (1992): "Mother matters: A fresh look at prenatal genetic testing." Issues *Repro Genet Engineer* 5(2):141-154.

Lippman A (1986): "Access to prenatal screening services: Who decides?" *Canad J Women Law* 1: 434-445.

Lippman A (1991): "Prenatal genetic testing and screening: Constructing needs and reinforcing inequities." *Amer J Law Med*, XVII (1 & 2):15-50.

Lippman A (1992): "Led (astray) by genetic maps: The cartography of the human genome and health care." *Soc Sci Med* 35(12):1469-76.

Lippman A, Brunger F (1991): "Constructing Down syndrome: Texts as Informants." *Santé Culture Health* VIII (1-2):109-131.

Lippman A, Wilfond BS (1992): "'Twice-Told tales': Stories about genetic disorders." *Amer J Hum Genet* 51:936-937.

Modell B, Kuliev AM (1991): "Services for thalassemia as a model for cost-benefit analysis of genetic services." *J Inherit Metab Dis* 14:640-651.

Payer L: *Medicine and culture.* New York: Viking, 1989.

Press NA, Browner CH (1993): "Collective fictions: Similarities in reasons for accepting MS FP screening among women of diverse ethnic and social class backgrounds." *Fetal Diagn* Ther 8 (Suppl):97-106.

Rosenberg CE (1992): Introduction. In: *Framing Disease: Studies in Cultural History,* Rosenberg CE, Golden J (eds). New Brunswick NJ: Rutgers Univ. Press.

Scutt JA (1991): "The politics of infertility 'counselling'": *Issues in Reprod and Genet Engineer* 4(3):251-256.

Shapiro R. "The human blueprint." Lecture, Science College Public Lecture Series, Concordia Univ., Montreal, 29 November 1990.

Spicker SF, Engelhardt HTJr (1984) "Causes and effects and side effects: Choosing between better and the best." *Health, Disease and Causal Explanation in Medicine,* NordenfeltL, Lindahl BIB (eds) Dordrecht: Reidel, p. 225.

Tesh SN (1988): *Hidden arguments: Political ideology and disease prevention policy.* New Brunswick, NJ: Rutgers Univ. Press.

NOTES

This paper derives from previously published material, especially articles in the American Journal of Law and Medicine, Issues in Reproductive and Genetic Engineering and Social Sciences and Medicine (see bibliography for details). Support for the research on which it is based has been provided by the Social Sciences and Humanities Research Council of Canada.

1 This is true only for some women having amniocentesis. With general population screening using alpha-fetoprotein or other chemical markers, women give samples for testing almost always without seeing a genetic counselor beforehand.

2 It is interesting that we seem to be quite comfortable rejecting prenatal diagnosis for sex selection because of our values (that females are no less valued than males), and recognize this as a value judgment, but reject any suggestion that value judgments imbue other decisions about eligibility for testing.

3 It is now to be offered to all pregnant women in Ontario.

4 An example of this is the tendency in the United States to see alcoholism as a "genetic" disorder among those living within its own borders but as a response to repressive sociopolitical conditions among those who live(d) in the former Soviet Union.

5 This claim is supported by reports of the unequal distribution in the use of other sophisticated biomedical testing programs, one recent example being the testing of newborn infants and their mothers for the presence of drugs which is selectively applied to poor and to Afro-American women in the United States.

6 Anti-smoking campaigns show this insofar as they have increased the difference in smoking rates between rich and poor as the former have been able to participate and thereby reduce usage while the latter have not.

3

CANADA AND THE GLOBAL CONTEXT OF THE NEW REPRODUCTIVE TECHNOLOGIES: A CAUTIONARY ESSAY

Sari Tudiver

"...it must be recognized that technology, by itself, cannot solve social and political problems."[1]

Over the past fifteen years I have spent considerable time pondering the many negative results of foreign aid policies of Western financial institutions and governments, including those of Canada. All too often, "development disasters" occurred when complex technologies were imposed without the collaboration and expertise of the people most directly affected, particularly the women. The short-term economic and political interests of those promoting the technologies determined development priorities without careful consideration of the possible long-term impacts. The consequences of inappropriate technologies affect not only local communities but, as in the case of pesticide misuse, come home to us in our morning coffee.[2]

As the new reproductive technologies become more common in Canada and in other parts of the world, I and others who have followed these trends have serious concerns about how these technologies are being developed both in Canada and internationally. In this chapter, I identify some of Canada's roles in a global political economy driven by private capital and state politics and link these to my concerns about increased commercialization of human life, reproduction and birthing, about genetic discrimination and about the potential uses of genetic manipulation for biological warfare. I argue that it is essential for consumer-driven, grass-roots groups to monitor how and by whom such technologies are researched, developed and applied and whose short-term and long-term interests are served. In order to ensure development appropriate to peoples' needs in Canada and internationally, we must take this critical information and formulate alternative visions, social policies and approaches to research.

CANADA IN GLOBAL ARENAS

The new reproductive technologies (NRTs) and the biotechnologies associated with them are part of lucrative and interlocking industries. They target genetic screening, prenatal diagnosis and gene therapy for women who are pregnant, hormonal contraceptives for women to prevent conception, and technologies such as *in vitro* fertilization (IVF), pre-implantation techniques and artificial insemination to try to overcome problems of infertility. Given the depth of feelings and the significance of reproduction in all cultures, societies and nation states, the world is truly their marketplace.

Canadian research and policies relating to NRTs are influenced by, and in turn affect, this global market. Canada is part of an international economic system in which capital, both Canadian and foreign, seeks resources, labour and markets in a global arena. Historically a major exporter of raw materials, Canada looks to increase the diversity of its industrial base and its exports. As biotechnologies and new reproductive technologies develop, Canadian policy makers and commercial interests, in collaboration with university-based scientists and the medical community are seeking shares in the world-wide research, development and trade of these potentially profitable sectors.

As a member of G-7, the United Nations and its various agencies, with representation to the World Bank, the International Monetary Fund (IMF) and GATT, and through participation in international scientific bodies, Canada allocates research and investment monies to projects pertaining to new reproductive technologies and biotechnologies and participates in related trade negotiations outside its borders. Through these fora, and as a signatory to a range of international covenants, conventions and agreements, Canada is also in a position to put forward any concerns about the development of these technologies.

Canada's foreign aid (approximately 2 percent of the federal budget and 0.43 percent of GNP in 1990) is carried out through a variety of bilateral, multilateral, non-governmental organizations (NGOs) and private sector channels. Through foreign aid Canada has reaped considerable prestige internationally and built up trade links with particular countries. Providing health aid dollars places Canada in a position to support or limit particular types of initiatives in recipient or "partner" countries. Thus, depending upon Canadian interests and policies, Canada can influence the host country and other donors to develop an infrastructure of rural primary health care facilities and wells for clean water, or finance large urban hospitals that offer IVF services.

The long-term and unexpected consequences of the Green Revolution (a movement during the 1960s and '70s to promote the application of new agricultural technologies designed to produce higher yields) — costly imports of agrochemicals, degradation of land and water due to pesticides and flooding, decline in genetic diversity of seeds and the control of new technologies by elites — led to greater dependence of Third World countries on the West and did little to ameliorate ill health and poverty.[3] The applications of other technologies to cultures and settings where they proved inappropriate, even disastrous, are well documented. Government, private capital and researchers bear moral and legal responsibilities to carefully evaluate the social implications of particular technologies and the potential effects on the health and safety of Canadians and other consumers. Considerable study and evaluation should precede the export and transfer of technologies, to determine whether in fact such technologies address significant, known health and social needs in other countries. In the development and application of new reproductive technologies, it is crucial to take direction from the poor, particularly poor women, about their priorities for health and other forms of development.

THE DEBT CRISIS AND ITS IMPLICATIONS FOR NRTS

The debt crisis is now a critical determining feature of international economic relations. Countries have reduced spending on health and social services, though rarely on military budgets, to pay massive interest on loans. As countries defaulted on payments, the IMF, World Bank and Western donor countries have instituted structural adjustment policies. To qualify for further aid or loans, Third World governments must devalue their currencies, reduce barriers to foreign investment, increase exports, freeze wages, raise food prices, and intensify efforts for family planning, among other conditions. Canadian aid policies officially support structural adjustment programs of the World Bank and IMF.

However, despite massive infusions of aid, there is a net outflow of resources from the South. According to UNICEF, since the early 1980s, the Third World pays the First World approximately $27 billion more than it receives in aid every year. U.N. data document that the number of absolute poor in the world has doubled over the past decade from 500 million to one billion and the gap between rich and poor has widened. The majority experience pressure on salaries, on the social services that they do have and on living standards generally.

People react to economic crises and to falling standards of living in a variety of ways. The poor, small business sector and professionals may be drawn into activities that were previously antithetical to their moral values and family structures. The poor, having no labour power to sell, sell their bodies, their future or life itself. Those better off exploit the demand for such products from national and international markets. These take a number of forms:

 * Children are sold for international adoption, as in Rumania, or parts of Latin America. Social workers and lawyers become brokers in this often questionable or illegal trade.

 * Within countries, both North and South, poor women are drawn to serve as "surrogates" for middle and upper income women.[4]

* In some countries (e.g. India, Singapore, Colombia), individuals sell their organs for human transplants.[5]

* There are mounting allegations that women, men and young children (e.g street children) from Central and South America and Asia, are kidnapped and killed so their organs and tissues may be used in their home countries and in North America, Europe and the Middle East, where there are not enough organs to meet the demand.[6]

Based on what is known about coercion and violence against women and children in all countries and documented through such agencies as the United Nations Commission on Modern Forms of Slavery, these practices must be acknowledged and addressed. If the markets for such products grow and people continue to experience severe economic hardships, there will be increasing pressure to secure embryos, eggs, sperm, fetal tissue and organs for a range of commercial and research purposes through whatever channels possible. Some Third World countries may become specialized in such products, part of a new international division of labour. This trade epitomizes practices and attitudes that presume Third World peoples to be inferior and "worth less" than those of Western countries that exploit their economic vulnerability.

Canadians need to question current government support for structural adjustment policies and major cuts to overseas development assistance which contribute to worsening economic conditions in Third World countries and which move away from earlier stated objectives to help achieve self-reliance in the poorest countries and enhance the status of women.[7] Specifically, Canadians also need to ask about the global implications of research and development of NRTs. For example, what are the sources of tissue and body parts used for research and commercial products in Canada and in other countries? Is it possible to have safeguards against illegal markets? Can we ethically proceed with research and commercial developments in Canada without asking about this first, rather than later? How can Canada play a key role through the United Nations and other agencies to document and stop violent practices? How can the transfer of appropriate technologies that meet local needs be assured?

These questions become even more pressing when we review the record of the international pharmaceutical industry and its crucial role in the research and development of reproductive technologies and biotechnologies.

THE INTERNATIONAL PHARMACEUTICAL INDUSTRY: CRITICAL PERSPECTIVES

The pharmaceutical industry emerged as a major power-broker in the post World War II period, stimulated by wartime research in the chemical industry. It expanded in a climate of optimism about scientific progress and few government controls and has remained a highly profitable industrial sector.[8] Since the mid-1980s, the worldwide industry reflects a number of characteristics and trends:

* The Industry is highly concentrated. While about 10,000 companies worldwide produce drugs, approximately 80 percent of the world's shipment of pharmaceutical products has been supplied by the largest 100 corporations.[9] In 1992, four major companies — Merck, Bristol-Myers Squibb, American Home Products and Eli Lilly — represented over one third of the total industry volume.[10] In Canada, transnational corporations control approximately 85 percent of the domestic market, a profile similar to many Third World countries. Decisions about what to research, produce and where are highly centralized. National governments may have little influence over such decisions; local communities, none at all.

* The Industry is diversified. The late 1960s and 1970s witnessed mergers and takeovers among many pharmaceutical and chemical companies. Through subsidiaries and branch plants around the world, most of the large pharmaceutical corporations produce a wide range of products in addition to drugs: agrochemicals, seeds, plastics, paints, cosmetics, veterinary and household products. In the early 1990s, many companies began moving into new products based on research in biotechnologies.

* Women constitute a large target group for research and marketing of pharmaceutical products. As primary care-givers to children, partners, aging parents or other relatives, women everywhere are major buyers and consumers of over-the-counter medications and prescription drugs. They are the sole users of a wide range of reproductive drugs and devices, fertility drugs, and estrogen replacement therapy promoted for long-term treatment of symptoms of menopause and for osteoporosis. Women are also major targets for mood-altering drugs, such as minor tranquilizers and anti-depressants, prescribed to persons experiencing anxiety, tension, nervousness and sleeplessness.[11]

A substantive literature documents the worrisome connection between women and pharmaceutical use: drugs, such as minor tranquilizers, are overprescribed to women; many drugs and devices, such as thalidomide, DES, and the Dalkon Shield IUD, have been marketed without adequate testing for long-term risks and under false claims of safety and efficacy. Western and Third World governments have been lax in the review process resulting in harm to women and children. Victims have had to organize to obtain information and secure recompense from hostile corporations and governments. Women have had little influence over decisions pertaining to research taken by the industry. They have been portrayed in stereotypic, often demeaning, sexist ads.

* The industry continues to produce many unnecessary and irrational products, such as skin lighteners, tonics and psychotropics, spending huge budgets on dubious advertising to promote them, despite urgent needs for affordable essential drugs. Many companies take advantage of lax regulations in some Third World countries to market drugs and devices not approved in countries where standards are more stringent and to promote licensed drugs for use beyond those for which they were approved or as over-the-counter products.[12]

* In Western and Third World countries, the pharmaceutical industry has lobbied governments to limit regulatory controls, such as requirements for drug testing. In Canada, they have also fought successfully for longer patent protection on brand name products.

THE PHARMACEUTICAL INDUSTRY, BIOTECHNOLOGY AND NRTS

Biotechnology brings revolutionary changes in processes and products and the capabilities to transform the genetic make-up of plants, animals and humans. The gene revolution allows for a "dematerialization of production," reducing the scale, energy input and volume of materials processed.[13] In the late 1980s and early 1990s, the large pharmaceutical/chemical companies have bought up or linked with small, research-intensive biotechnology companies which needed access to capital and larger facilities.[14] Commercial developments of these technologies by them lead to major economic and social restructuring with global implications.

Industries which had gone offshore are returning to the core countries, leaving Third World countries even more dependent on their agricultural exports. But as a result of biotechnologies applied to agriculture, many Third World agricultural products will no longer be in demand. There will be a new international division of labour, in which specialist products might come from single installations, and operations might move readily from one region or country to another, depending on the needs of capital. Third World governments will be increasingly desperate for investment and may embrace industries and research that reflect the priorities of Western countries, rather than their own. They may bring risks to public health and to the environment from genetically engineered organisms.[15]

From what we know about the transnational pharmaceutical industry, some trends pertaining to NRTs can be identified:

* Developments in biotechnology, such as the production of reproductive hormones in bacteria or DNA probes, will facilitate *in vitro* fertilization, embryo freezing and prenatal diagnosis.[16]

* The pharmaceutical/chemical/biotechnology industry will develop products and processes that promise major profits. For example, drug companies are moving into new biotech products in

cosmetics, estimated at multi-billion dollar markets annually. There are also vast commercial implications for genetic screening. As well, many researchers own stock and so have vested interests in their company's operations and policies. These may conflict with research priorities identified by government or consumers and with a critical review of their own research findings or those of their colleagues.

* Third World women will continue to be used as test subjects for many drugs and procedures such as superovulatory drugs, genetic screening tests, vaccines and IVF. Since legislation and research protocols are lax in many countries, researchers will go where they can more easily advance their work. Governments will welcome such research and ensure women are available. As with hormonal contraceptives, research into long-term risks of drugs and procedures will not be carried out prior to use of the technologies on women; rather, women and children will become research subjects who may be monitored for long-term health effects.

Consolidation among major, Western-based transnationals will likely continue, but may take some new directions. For example, given the profits to be made in the application of biotechnology to food-processing, major food companies may merge with pharmaceutical companies. Pharmaceutical and life insurance companies may consolidate as part of a "life technology industry." In one possible scenario, tissue samples at birth will be stored in banks; person-specific drugs may be developed from body tissue and multiplied in plants or animals; companies might have rights over tissues and provide health services. The processing of genetic information will be key in such an industry.[17]

PATENTS

In the U.S., Canada and many other Western countries, protection is permitted on novel seeds, plants and plant tissue cultures. Transnationals control supplies of seeds to Africa and Southeast Asia and limit the possibilities for indigenous experimentation and control over agriculture. Third World countries that were the sources of many of the original seed varieties are losing their genetic plant diversity. Moreover, they have provided the folk medicinal plants and knowledge for an estimated one-quarter of the value of the present pharmaceutical industry, but have received no recompense through patents.

Since 1981, the U.S. has moved speedily towards legal recognition of the right to patent a live organism, where some of its properties were deemed to be the result of invention. In 1987, the U.S. Patent Office issued a ruling that patents could be extended to animals that were subject to genetic manipulation. Since 1988, there have been increasing numbers of patents granted for genetically altered animals.

This commercialization of biotechnology and genetic manipulation will proceed rapidly, supported by the legal recognition of patents to the products and processes of biotechnology.[18] Already in the U.S., hundreds of human cell lines listed with the American Type Culture Collection are under patent or the subject of patent applications.[19]

U.S. and Australian proposals in the GATT Trade-Related Intellectual Property (GATT TRIP) negotiations are demanding that plant, animal and microbial biological products and processes be subject to universal patent monopoly.[20] Contracting parties would be obliged to adopt national legislation granting such rights to foreign enterprises. Massive royalty payments would increase from Third World countries to the U.S. alone by about \$43-61 billion per year — roughly equal to the annual debt repayments.

While the proposals make no direct reference to patenting life forms, they argue non-exclusion, and resist wording that clearly excludes people. This is largely because research is proceeding which breaks down the boundaries between species and biological kingdoms, and for example, allows human genes to be inserted into mice, pigs, sheep and plants. The ability to patent such new life forms might be threatened if "humans" could not be patentable. The aim of the GATT TRIP negotiations is to ensure control by Western industries over the microbial, plant and animal genetic resources in Third World countries, which provide crucial raw materials for biotechnology and genetic engineering. In addition to the wide range of moral and ethical issues raised globally, Third World countries stand to lose in terms of economic returns and negotiating power if biological materials are included in the GATT TRIPS.

Patenting life forms involves the collaboration of Western industrialized states, including Canada, with corporate and scientific interests to consolidate economic and political power. The dangerous illusion that some can "own for profit" knowledge about human life and reproduction has serious practical consequences.

DOMINANT RESEARCH PARADIGMS: TWO BRIEF EXAMPLES

Current international development policies and the practices of science are rooted in the assumptions and practices of mercantile capitalism, colonial expansion and militarism, and in Western attitudes that devalued women and people of colour at least from the 17th century on.[21] A number of characteristics define this paradigm:

* It is objectivist: the language used turns experience and pain into an object of study, divorced from its context and assumes it to be reality, not itself laden with values.

* It is characterized by "power-over" — whether the conquest of nature, the enemy, turning people into slaves, cheap labour, or sources of sperm and ova.

* It is arrogant: in science, this is reflected in the belief that all things can be known. In development, the arrogance has a long history as racism, proselytizing, the degradation of women and forms of paternalism, such as the transfer of Western technologies with the assumption that Western ways are best for others.

* It is enamoured of "quick-fix" technological solutions to complex social and environmental problems.

* There is a tendency to fragment and compartmentalize fields of study in science. In development this is reflected in the fragmentation of aid.

* It is common for scientists to deny responsibility for the consequences of their research or actions. Governments and development agencies responsible for projects are rarely accountable for the failures of aid.

* Sexism and the use of violent sexual language and imagery has a long history in science ("the rape of nature") and is well documented for the military and its weapons.[22] Until very recently, in development initiatives, women have been devalued and rendered invisible and the violence against them ignored.[23]

Mapping the human genome and research into biological warfare reflect many of the features of this dominant paradigm promoted by the State and corporate capital. They are useful examples to illustrate how reproductive and genetic technologies are being promoted before their implications for present and future generations are widely understood.

HUMAN GENOME MAPPING

Research directed towards mapping the human genome is proceeding in a number of countries and has important implications for development of the new reproductive technologies. Drawing genetic maps and linking a vast array of disorders to specific genes and DNA sequences provide the basis for genetic screening of populations, including prenatal screening. IVF and other reproductive technologies, gene therapy, adoption, surrogacy or not having children at all, may be the ways people identified as carriers of particular disease genes try to avoid having children at risk of particular disabilities.

Major initiatives pertaining to human genome mapping are underway in Canada, the U.S., England and Japan, with some projects in France, Italy and other Western European countries. Research is supported by government departments, government-funded institutions and by private companies. Smaller scale research is being carried out in Brazil, Argentina and India. There is interest in the results of the research for addressing specific genetic diseases common to their populations on the part of Mexico, other Latin American countries and some African countries.[24]

Over the past five years, there have been efforts to coordinate international work in human genome mapping. The major examples have been those of the Human Genome Organization (HUGO), an international body of scientists attempting to facilitate mapping efforts, share data and promote interest in commercial applications of the mapping work. More recently, the Human Genome Diversity Project, funded by the U.S. National Institute of Health and linked to HUGO, has begun a campaign to take blood, tissue and hair samples from hundreds of "endangered" indigenous communities around the world before they die out.[25]

The human genome mapping projects raise a number of concerns:[26]

* They involve large allocations of resources, drawn from sources that might support research directed to more immediate social and medical needs in countries of the North and South.[27] Because of strong scientific and commercial pressures, foreign aid monies that might have been used for public health measures that address many of the causes of disabilities may be diverted to support genome mapping and sampling.

* The research has resulted in techniques for genetic diagnosis and DNA-based identification of diseases and disabilities that could not be predicted before. For a majority of these, however, there are no therapies. This widens the gap between diagnosis and treatment and raises numerous ethical and social issues about creating and then addressing people's anxieties about illness or potential illness and stigmas. Some researchers acknowledge the unforeseen anguish and complications resulting from decisions to be tested for conditions such as Huntington disease which appear later in life.[28]

* Detailed personal information is generated through genetic screening which is sought by insurance companies, employers and State agencies. There are increased opportunities for genetically based discrimination.[29]

* Undue emphasis is placed on the role of the gene and gene sequencing in human behaviour, while the complex interactions between genes and organisms and the social/cultural environment are minimized. In looking for genetic components of diseases, illness is decontextualized. Environmental causes are downplayed and attention drawn away from necessary political changes. The majority of disabilities do not have genetic causes.[30] The "geneticization of human behavior" offers a paradigm compatible with social/eugenic abuses.[31]

* As researchers try to determine human genetic diversity and similarities, Third World peoples and ethnic minorities in Western countries are perceived as objects of human genome research. As one investigator comments, "Developing nations have a crucial role in the human genome project, as the mapping of human disease genes depends on having large families. These nations can provide the requisite pedigrees for mapping."[32] While researchers often note that special precautions must be taken to protect the confidentiality, autonomy and dignity of all individuals and families involved in research studies, experiences with other health research on Third World populations indicate that this can be difficult to achieve in practice.

Given that mapping and commercialization of the human genome appear to be increasing in scope internationally, it is crucial for Canadians to determine the current status of such research in Canada, including the nature and scale of government and other sources of funding. The ethical and social implications of the human genome projects, including the impacts of projects in Third World contexts, must be subject to public review. Why will human genetic material be stored? Who will or might have access to stored genetic material and where will collections be located? How will safeguards to individual privacy be assured? The profits, benefits and risks of such research have not been subject to broad discussion. So far, indigenous peoples' organizations and international consumer organizations with interests in such issues have not been included in project planning or negotiations.

BIOLOGICAL WEAPONS AND NEW REPRODUCTIVE AND GENETIC TECHNOLOGIES

The Biological Weapons Convention outlaws the development, possession and stockpiling of biological weapons for offensive military purposes. It allows research, development and possession for defensive and other "peaceful purposes." The most recent review of the Convention in 1986 strengthened it with improved measures for verification and for making it part of the civil legal code of each country. Serious concerns remain since it is almost impossible to distinguish defensive from offensive weapons.

Considerable money is spent by the military on biological weapons research, including research on plague, anthrax, smallpox, malaria, meningitis and other largely "Third World" diseases. U.S. data show a ten-fold increase in this area from 1976-1986, despite ratification of the 1972 Biological Weapons Convention. Russia, Britain, Iraq, Israel and numerous other countries engage in research. There are, no doubt, specific regions (e.g. crop areas) in Western and Third World countries used for testing such research, although government secrecy makes this difficult to determine.[33]

Genetic manipulation opens up new possibilities in biological weapons. Quantities of virulent agents targeted to crops, animals or humans can be produced that are resistant to antibiotics or pesticides. Vaccines can be developed to protect the troops of one country against agents directed to enemies. It will be possible to target specific ethnic/racial groups based on genotype differences; mutagenic agents would act on the germ-line and affect later generations. DNA probes and research related to genetic screening are relevant to research on biological weapons.

Given the global implications of biological weapons research, it is crucial to determine the specific links between research and development of new reproductive and genetic technologies and development of biological weapons. What technologies are particularly relevant to biological weapons research?[34] What is the status of biological weapons research in Canada? Do Canadian researchers in universities, companies and the military, carry out such research for the Canadian military or under contract to the U.S.? The secrecy surrounding such research during World War II and in the post-war period suggests that current research may be equally difficult to confirm.[35]

As a party to the Biological Weapons Convention, are there specific ways in which Canada can intervene to ensure greater public scrutiny over the international monitoring process? Are there ways to ensure that research pertaining to new reproductive and genetic technologies is not used for military purposes?

ALTERNATE PARADIGMS

The human genome project and biological weapons research represent the mainstream paradigm. Are there other ways?

Alternative paradigms could be based on very different, contrary principles and practices. Advocates could stress the interrelationships between subject and object and recognize that technologies are not neutral but developed and applied by particular interest groups in the exercise of power. They could find ways to truly share power, resources and expertise between countries of the North and South and to democratize decision-making about the allocation of resources. Priority could be given to researching longer term, sustainable solutions appropriate to peoples' needs at local and regional levels.

Alternative paradigms appear at the margins and are evident in the understandings gained from aboriginal and other non-Western cultures, from the experiences and insights of many women, victims, recipients of aid, from those who care about the environment. How effectively such advocates educate, communicate and work with others to form broad and powerful social movements will determine whether alternative paradigms displace what we now know as the dominant forms.

Non-governmental organizations, women's health and consumer networks such as Health Action International, the Seeds Action Network, the International Organization of Consumer Unions and the Latin American and Caribbean Women's Health Network, play key roles monitoring global trends in the pharmaceutical and biotechnology industries and work towards important changes in practices. The Feminist International Network of Resistance to Reproductive and Genetic Engineering (FINRRAGE) offers one model of international cooperation and collaboration among feminist scholars, researchers and activists. Women from over twenty-five countries of the North and South are involved in monitoring developments in reproductive technologies and genetic manipulation, debating and analyzing the social, legal, and ethical dimensions of these technologies.[36] Needed are discussions addressing potential benefits of screening or gene therapy in treatment of specific medical conditions, useful applications of biotechnology in Western and Third World contexts and models of collaboration between Western and indigenous science.

Many non-governmental organizations have crucial insights to offer based on decades of experience working in Third World countries in reproductive health and in the transfer of technologies. NGOs have mostly attempted to address basic needs in agriculture, health, literacy and economic development, but have learned, in the process, about macro-economic and political conditions that facilitate or block sustainable development. Successful projects have been ones in which local people determined their priorities; which applied technologies appropriate to local resources; and where the sophisticated and varied knowledge of local farmers, healers and other workers — who are often women — is equally weighted with Western science.

As many Canadian NGOs become clearer about the kinds of approaches needed for long-term sustainability and are working towards more equitable relations with international partners, they are losing ground within the Canadian aid arena. This is reflected in declining government dollars to NGOs, reorganizations within The Canadian International Development Agency (CIDA) and strong government emphasis on business sector initiatives in foreign aid. These competing paradigms to aid will affect whether Canada moves rapidly to take advantage of any commercial development internationally in NRTs or opts for the technologies to be evaluated more cautiously.

As a cultural phenomenon, biotechnology, genetic manipulation and the new reproductive technologies suggest new frontiers about the nature of life and the art of the possible. At the same time, corporate capital, governments, researchers, patent negotiators and commissions of inquiry limit our vision by organizing and controlling development of these technologies in ways that consolidate rather than share their knowledge and power. We must formulate alternate visions and approaches using the considerable expertise of the women's health and other progressive social movements in Canada and internationally to determine health research priorities and social policies. Can alternate loci of control over particular technologies be developed? If so, how?

Reproduction should be about respect, love, continuity, caring and compassion; about supporting and accepting differences. The majority of research in new reproductive technologies is unlikely to enhance these values. Nor will it eradicate poverty and violence against women and children, major causes of disability. More likely, such research and technologies will deepen the gap between rich and poor by commercializing life and reproduction, creating new environmental hazards and iatrogenic illnesses and drawing resources and political attention away from needed social change. These are not sustainable approaches to human and social development.

The allocation of research monies to specific reproductive technologies, genome mapping and military "defence" rather than to other social needs must be broadly discussed and debated in Canada. Government, corporate capital, scientific interest groups and the military must be accountable to those who ultimately fund and experience the effects of current practices and policies. Research and its applications must take place in a context of caution and humility to ensure the least harm and hopefully some benefits to current and future generations. The consequences of haste and arrogance lie beyond *Jurassic Park*.

NOTES

1 Colin Norman, *The God That Limps: Science and Technology in the Eighties* (New York: W.W. Norton) 1981, p.186.

2 Some key works include: Cheryl Payer, *The World Bank - A Critical Analysis* (New York: Monthly Review Press) 1982; Barbara Rogers, *The Domestication of Women: Discrimination in Developing Societies* (New York: St. Martin's Press) 1980; and Catherine Overholt, et al., eds. *Gender Roles in Development Projects* (West Hartford: Kumarian Press) 1985.

3 For a cogent review of the impacts of the Green Revolution and of the application of biotechnologies to food production see Vandana Shiva, *Staying Alive: Women, Ecology and Development* (London: Zed Books Ltd) 1988, Chapter 5.

4 See chapters by Eichler and Sherwin.

5 See B. Dickens, "Ethics, Justice and Commerce in Transplantation: A Global Issue" (Ottawa, 20-24 August, 1989). *International Digest of Health Legislation*, 1990, 41 (1). International Conference sponsored by Health and Welfare Canada with the Transplantation Society. Kidney purchases from unrelated live donors were confirmed.

6 These allegations were made by Dr. Rosalie Bertell at the Conference on Ethics, Justice and Commerce in Transplantation: A Global Issue in Ottawa, 20-24 August, 1989. She called for a universal prohibition of human organ sales. *International Digest of Health Legislation*, 1990, 41 (1), pp. 179-182 reviews the conference. See also Janice Raymond, "Children for organ export?" *Reproductive and Genetic Engineering*, Vol. 2, No. 3, 1989, pp. 237-245; and J. Raymond, "The international traffic in women: Women used in systems of surrogacy and reproduction," *Reproductive and Genetic Engineering*, Vol. 2, No. 1, 1989, pp. 51-57. E. Yoxen and B. Hyde, *The Social Impact of Biotechnology*, Luxembourg: Office for Official Publications of the European Communities, 1987, p.39 also refer to a black market in organs.

7 Canadian overseas development assistance was cut by close to $1.75 billion in 1990 over a five year period and in 1991 by another $1.6 billion over the next five year period. Government policies continue to erode bilateral aid and aid through Canadian NGOs to poor countries, while seeking new Third World markets for Canadian private investors. For a recent review of trends in aid see, Clyde Sanger, "Out of Africa," *Canadian Forum*, July/August, 1993, pp. 18-23.

8 Ongoing analyses of trends in the pharmaceutical industry can be gleaned from critical sources such as "Another Development in Pharmaceuticals", Special Issue of *Development Dialogue*, No. 2, 1985; "Molecules and Markets: A Survey of Pharmaceuticals," *The Economist*, February 7, 1987; World Health Organization, *The World Drug Situation* (Geneva: WHO) 1988; and regular Standard and Poor's Industry Surveys and trade publications.

9 Source: C. Fowler, E. Lachkovics, P. Mooney and H. Shand, "The Laws of Life: Another Development and the New Biotechnologies." *Development Dialogue*. 1988: 1-2. Dag Hammarskjold Foundation. *Uppsala*. pp 161 (1985 data). This superb volume summarizes international developments in biotechnology and links between biotechnlogy and pharmaceutical companies.

10 Standard and Poor's Industry Surveys, *Health Care*, August 20, 1992, p. H18.

11 The multi-billion dollar contraceptive industry includes barrier methods, an increasing array of hormonal contraceptives - oral contraceptives, injectables, implants, and IUDs which release synthetic hormones. For a good overview of these issues, see Kathleen McDonnell, *Adverse Effects: Women and the Pharmaceutical Industry*. (Toronto: Women's Press) 1986.

12 Since its formation in 1981, Health Action International, a coalition of health professionals and consumers has monitored and documented these practices internationally. See for example, Dianna Melrose, *Bitter Pills: Medicines and the Third World Poor* (Oxford: OXFAM UK), 1982; Andrew Chetley, *A Healthy Business? World Health and the Pharmaceutical Industry* (London: Zed Books) 1990; Michael L. Tan, *Dying for Drugs: Pill Power and Politics in the Philippines* (Quezon City: Health Action Information Network) 1988.

13 Yoxen and Hyde, op. cit., p. 11.

14 The growth of the biotech firms has been rapid. By 1990 there were over 1000 companies engaged primarily in biotechnology. Just under half are in the U.S., many in Japan and Western Europe. Some companies are in Brazil, India, Republic of Korea and Taiwan. U.N. Centre on Transnational Corporations, Transnational Corporations and the Transfer of New and Emerging Technologies to Developing Countries (New York: United Nations) 1990.

15 Biotech agricultural research is occurring in Brazil, Argentina, Mexico, India, Malaysia, Pakistan, the Philippines, Thailand and in several African countries. Third World countries are increasingly pressed by the West to adopt or experiment with various biotechnology industries because they are "clean" environmentally and will not further contribute to global environmental degradation. Third World countries may provide a large testing ground for products and industries. (Personal Communication, Senior Advisor, United Nations Non-governmental Liaison Service, New York, June 25, 1991.)

16 Yoxen and Hyde, op. cit., p.33.

17 I am indebted to Pat Mooney of the Rural Advancement Foundation International for his insights into these trends.

18 U.N. Centre on Transnational Corporations, Transnational Corporations and the Transfer of New and Emerging Technologies to Developing Countries (New York: United Nations) 1990. ST/CTC/98.

19 The U.S. National Institute of Health applied for patents on genes and DNA fragments found in the human brain, despite not knowing what functions these served. While the U.S. Patent Office rejected the applications, the NIH scientists plan to reapply. RAFI Communiqué, 1993.

20 This section draws from Rural Advancement Foundation International paper, "GATTLORE: The North's Strategy to Patent Biological Diversity in GATT (TRIPS)," 1990.

21 For some basic feminist critiques of scientific ideologies and practices, including military research, see: Carolyn Merchant, *The Death of Nature: Women, Ecology and the Scientific Revolution* (San Francisco: Harper and Row) 1983 and 1990; Nancy Tuana, ed., *Feminism and Science* (Bloomington: Indiana Univerity Press) 1989; Brian Easlea, *Fathering the Unthinkable: Masculinity, Scientists and the Nuclear Arms Race* (London: Pluto Press) 1983.

22 See both Merchant and Easlea, op. cit.

23 See Gita Sen and Caren Grown, *Development Crises, and Alternative Visions: Third World Women's Perspectives* (New York: Monthly Review Press) 1987.

24 For a clear and generally favorable overview of the status of genome research at the end of the 1980s, see Congress of the U.S. Office of Technology Assessment, *Mapping Our Genes. Genome Projects: How Big, How Fast?* (Washington, D.C.: U.S. G.P.O.) April, 1988. The report contains a good summary of social and ethical considerations and issues pertaining to transfer of technology. Canadian funding for Human Genome Project research was approximately $22 million in 1992.

25 Referred to as "isolates of historic interest," or "IHIs" in their proposal. Rural Advancement Foundation International (RAFI) Communiqué, 1993.

26 See also the chapters by Lippman.

27 See OTA study, Appendix A on costs of U.S. programs. The Human Genome Diversity Project estimates that gathering samples from relatively accessible populations over the first five year period will cost between $23 and $35 million dollars. RAFI Communiqué, May, 1993, 2.

28 OTA, 1988, p. 83. See Jerry E. Bishop and Michael Waldholz, *Genome* (New York: Touchstone Books) 1991, chapters 13, 14 and 15 for a discussion of the complex issues raised by "predictive medicine."

29 For a useful summary of the critiques see Council for Responsible Genetics, "Position Paper on Genetic Discrimination," and "Position Paper on Human Genome Initiative," *Issues in Reproductive and Genetic Engineering*, Vol. 3, No. 3, 1990. For a good discussion and specific recommendations pertaining to legal reforms and rights to privacy in the Canadian context, see The Privacy Commissioner of Canada, *Genetic Testing and Privacy*, (Ottawa: Minister of Supply and Services Canada) 1992.

30 Council on Human Genetics, "Position Paper on Human Genome Initiative," p. 293.

31 See Abby Lippman, "Prenatal Genetic Testing and Screening: Constructing Needs and Reinforcing Inequities," *American Journal of Law and Medicine*, Vol. XVII Nos. 1&2, 1991.

32 N. Wexler. quoted in Z. Bankowski and A.M. Capron, eds., *Genetics, Ethics and Human Values: Human Genome Mapping, Genetic Screening and Gene Therapy. Proceedings of the XXIVth CIOMS Conference, Tokyo and Inuyama City, Japan,* July, 1990. CIOMS, Geneva, 1991. p.186.

33 See the discussion of biological warfare and weapons in David Suzuki and Peter Knudtson, *Genethics: The Ethics of Engineering Life* (Toronto: Stoddart Publishing) 1988, chapter 9; and Cary Fowler, Eva Lachkovics et al., op cit. pp. 194-211; and Richard Novick and Seth Shulman, "New Forms of Biological Warfare?" *geneWATCH*, Vol. 6, No. 6, 1990.

34 Very little has been researched specifically on the links to NRTs. For example, a NATO seminar focused on IVF in 1984. For what purposes? See Linda Bullard, "Killing Us Softly: Toward a Feminist Analysis of Genetic Engineering," in P. Spallone and D. Steinberg, *Made to Order: The Myth of Reproductive and Genetic Progress* (Oxford: Pergamon Press), 1987.

35 See John Bryden, *Deadly Allies: Canada's Secret War 1937-1947* (Toronto: McClelland and Stewart), 1989.

36 FINRRAGE generates quality research and analysis through an excellent journal, *Issues in Reproductive and Genetic Engineering*, conferences and reports. Discussions reveal contrasting approaches to questions of individual and collective rights, bioethics and disability. The possible long-term impacts of genetic screening and genetic engineering are assessed.

4

IS THE ISSUE CHOICE?

Judy Rebick

I have been an activist in the pro-choice movement for more than ten years. From 1981 to 1988 I was probably the most visible female spokesperson for the pro-choice movement in Canada. I believe that women's right to control our reproduction, including the right to abortion, is fundamental to women's equality.

Nevertheless, over the last few years I have come to question our self-appellation as the "pro-choice" movement. The struggle for abortion rights is and has always been a struggle of women to win control over our own bodies from the state and the church — and in some circumstances from the men in our lives. It is about autonomy and self-determination. The use of the term "choice" developed as a powerful way to explain that what we wanted was the right to make our own decisions. In supporting abortion rights, we explain, you do not have to agree with abortion or even be willing to choose it as an option for yourself, but rather be willing to recognize someone else's right to make that choice. Because freedom of choice is such a strong value in liberal democratic society, the pro-choice argument became the most successful argument in our repertory and we came to rely on it more and more.

While we may have won popular support on the basis of the pro-choice argument, we did not win the struggle to legalize abortion on this argument. In fact, in the majority judgment in the Morgentaler case, Chief Justice Dickson based his decision on a different argument, that women had the right to control their own bodies.

Moreover by focusing on choice we have created the mistaken impression that feminism is about freedom of choice in all spheres. In the abortion fight, many women of colour, poor women and women with disabilities have argued that the choice slogan excluded them. They support abortion rights but don't feel that they really have freedom of choice. A poor black woman who decides on a abortion may do so because she simply cannot afford to feed another child, not because she doesn't want to have one. Not much of a choice. Our response in the pro-choice movement was to talk about giving women true choices and then incorporating other demands for women's equality, such as employment equity, an end to violence against women, etc., into the choice lexicon. At a recent NAC conference, a young woman defined feminism as fighting for women to have more choices in their lives.

But is feminism really about freedom of choice in all spheres? I think not. Feminism is about achieving equality for all women. In a class and race-divided society, freedom of choice for one woman can mean virtual slavery for another, for example contract motherhood. By turning one argument for abortion rights into the very definition of the movement itself, I believe we have identified feminism with the civil libertarian notion of the supremacy of individual rights. The idea that individual choice is the most important social value is not particularly feminist. In fact, in a society of unequal power, an emphasis on individual choice alone usually gives those with power the only real choices. Feminism seeks to change the power structures in society, to empower those with less power, women, racial minorities, the poor, etc. This can often conflict with individual choice on a given issue.

It was during the debate on New Reproductive Technologies that I really began to question the focus on choice as the issue. When NAC took the position for a moratorium on new IVF clinics and a ban on surrogacy, we got hammered in the media for the contradiction between our position on abortion and our position on IVF. "Why is NAC for choice in deciding not to have children but against choice in deciding to have children?" they demanded. In response we argued that in the case of IVF the choice of an individual woman could be detrimental to women as a group and that we needed to look at the impact of IVF on the future of women's equality and reproduction and not just on the individual life of the woman. Some pro-choice activists said that this argument was a slippery slope that could lead to an anti-choice position on abortion as well. While I rejected that argument at the time, I think it has some merit. But the problem, I would submit, is not our position on NRTs but rather our accepting the appellation of pro-choice to define the abortion rights movement.

With a framework of controlling our bodies as women, feminist opposition to the new reproductive and genetic technologies is much clearer. These technologies are taking control of our reproduction out of our hands and perhaps eventually out of our bodies altogether and placing it in the hands of doctors and scientists. There is no question that IVF provides a solution for some infertile women who have strong desires to have a child. But if that solution puts many more women at risk, then is it a solution that the women's movement can support, however much we empathize with the plight of infertile women? While using the term "pro-choice" was important to winning the abortion debate, I am now convinced that the framework of our position on reproductive rights must be the right to control our bodies and reproduction rather than freedom of individual choice.

PART II

EUGENICS FROM THEN TO NOW

Eugenics. It's a "dirty" word, one we don't like to say; a practice we don't like to think occurs. But say it we must, and think about it too. And the chapters that follow do just this.

Eugenics, choosing who will be the parents of future generations and selecting who will be the members of these generations, took on its modern guise in the early years of this century when the genetic basis for the inheritance of familial characteristics was identified. Farmers and animal breeders eagerly adopted eugenic procedures for their attempts to improve their produce and livestock (Annette Burfoot). Eugenics quickly became the basis of Social Darwinism as political elites saw selective breeding of people as a way for science to manage what they considered intractible social problems. It gained subsequent infamy in the policies of Hitler's Germany (Lynn Glazier; Varda Burstyn). Subsequently, too, it has gained frightening dimensions as humans become the experimental models for developing ever new approaches to genetic manipulation, also known as "eugenics" (Gwynne Basen). As these papers so forcefully document, eugenics — or at least the thinking and values it encompasses — lives on.

And in this continued life, eugenics takes still other forms. Now it is not overt public policy so much as social custom and private practice that drive selection. Marketed as "choice" for the sex of one's child (Sunera Thobani), for having a child without some disability at birth (Maria Barile; Sandra Goundry and the CDRC), eugenics becomes more subtle. Some refer to this as "quality control," but others insist it is merely giving women who have long demanded the right to choose the number of children they will bear a parallel "right" with respect to the kind of children they will bear. But, as these three papers show most clearly, the latter is a fallacious, and not a merely superficial, position. It is a position, moreover, that enjoins feminists to search together for the common ground on which to reconsider "selective" abortion, abortion because of some characteristic of the fetus detected *in utero*.

This long-needed conversation, indeed a renewed assessment of the entire eugenic underpinning of the new reproductive and genetic technologies, is initiated thoughtfully by all the women writing in the pages that follow.

5

PLAYING GOD: MEDICAL ETHICS AND HISTORY'S FORGOTTEN LESSONS

Lynn Glazier

"The cattle car door slid open and the mass of people spilled out on the platform. My mother grabbed my twin sister and me by the hands. Somehow she hoped she could protect us by holding onto us," recalls Eva Mozes-Kor, a survivor of the experiments conducted on some 1500 sets of twins at Auschwitz from 1943 to 1945. "I looked around and everything looked very, very depressing. Grey. Tall barbed wires. I could see chimneys, I could smell the unbearable smell." That day her parents and two older sisters were sent to the gas chamber. The nine-year-old girls, Eva and her sister Miriam, became guinea pigs in Josef Mengele's laboratory.

The notorious "Angel of Death" is perhaps the most potent symbol of evil in the history of modern medicine. With a wave of his hand Mengele chose the fit and the unfit at the camp gates. The selection of who lived and who died was in effect a medical diagnosis. This is a symbol of a physician as someone who makes decisions about the value of human life.

The Third Reich was obsessed with twin research in its quest to unravel the nature-nurture dichotomy. Mengele was an ardent practitioner. His experiments on twins were senseless and diabolical — injecting lethal viruses, amputating and re-attaching limbs, performing skin and bone grafts without anesthetic. It was torture and murder, not science.

Yet Mengele's mentor and sponsor was the head of the prestigious Kaiser Wilhelm Institute of Anthropology in Berlin. Professor Otmar Von Verschuer resumed his scientific career after the war and became the head of genetics at the University of Munster. "Dr. Von Verschuer continues to this day to be a respected pioneer in the field of research on twins. His work in genetics has become part of the complex field of mapping the human genome. The command Mengele shouted on the rail platform of Auschwitz, 'Zwillinge heraus! Zwillinge heraustreten! (Twins out! Twins, step forward!) originated not with a deranged monster working in isolation, but with an internationally respected scientist who remains a cited authority in the field of genetics," writes William Seidelman in a 1989 paper on medicine's Nazi heritage published in the *International Journal of Health Services*. He is a leading Canadian authority on the legacy of Nazi medicine and a professor of family medicine at McMaster University.

The worst atrocities ever committed in the name of science were part of the efforts of the German biomedical establishment to "improve the species." Now, a half century later, science is promising a new and better way to benefit humankind. We are developing the sophisticated technology to reveal the very blueprint of biological imperfection which lies in our genes.

But what lesson is there in a discussion of torture and genocide in contemporary science? A consensus is emerging among bioethicists that Nazi doctors must not be dismissed as a mere aberration. They say it is appropriate to look at how reputable scientists got caught up in an ideology which did not begin with the Nazis and did not die with them. "Bioethics must be viewed from history," says the director of the Centre for Bioethics at the University of Minnesota, Arthur Caplan, "and it's one of the failings of current bioethical thinking that it's done with almost no attention to history."

That statement points to a very complex web of issues that is on the cutting edge of ethical debate in science and medicine today. Like Caplan, many bioethicists argue that the only meaningful discussion of biomedical ethics must take place in an historical context. The legacy of the past is all too relevant in today's scientific climate where anything seems possible and money dictates who benefits. Yet in our excitement about new technological advances — particularly in genetics — we have forgotten history's most important lessons about judging the value of human life. While science is in itself value-free, its application is not.

Research for the sake of science, not humanity, was the rule in much of the western world in the first half of the 20th century. The first international code of bioethics rose out of the ashes of the Holocaust. But almost as soon as the ten principles of the Nuremberg Code were written and the primacy of human rights in human experimentation was asserted, all was forgotten. It was only in response to the atrocities committed in the name of science in Nazi Germany that a new discipline in medicine evolved — ethics. But history tells us that the times we don't take ethics seriously are often when it matters most.

One of the most telling examples of this tunnel vision in the North American history of human experimentation is the infamous Tuskegee Study. Four hundred American black men suffering from syphilis were deliberately left untreated for decades (even after the effectiveness of penicillin was established in the early 1940s) to study the effects of the disease.

Most of the subjects were not told they had syphilis — only that they had "bad blood" — and none knew they were guinea pigs. The study ran from 1932 to 1972. It began before the Holocaust, continued through it, and after the Nuremberg Code and its entrenchment of the concept of voluntary consent. This episode in the history of medical science is not mentioned in bioethics textbooks.

In Canada, the CIA sponsored brainwashing experiments on more than fifty psychiatric patients without their consent at the Allan Memorial Institute in Montreal during the 1950s and 1960s. Dr. Ewan Cameron subjected patients to repeated electro-shocks and drug induced sleep (in one case for as long as eighty-six days) intended to wipe the mind clean, so that new "healthy" messages could be imprinted by psychic driving experiments where subjects were forced to listen to hypnotic tapes for days on end.

The patients came into the Institute with problems like post-partum depression and nervous conditions. Many survivors of these experiments were left with permanent memory loss, chronic depression and migraines. Dr. Cameron was not seen as a "mad" scientist at the time. During his career he was the president of the Quebec, Canadian, American and World Psychiatric Associations.

Robert Jay Lifton, psychiatrist and author of *The Nazi Doctors: Medical Killing and the Psychology of Genocide* stated in an affidavit filed in the United States on behalf of Canadians suing the CIA: "These procedures were experimental and deviated from customary pyschiatric therapies in use during the 1950s." He added that Dr. Cameron failed "to maintain the ethically required distinction between research and healing" and that the experiments "closely paralleled the techniques of 'thought reform' or 'brainwashing' used in Chinese prisons." It was not until survivors started coming forward with their horror stories in the last ten years that Dr. Cameron's work was censured.

That is the pattern of modern science — when we look to the past for guidance, it is the triumphs and successes of the previous generation, not the blunders, we acknowledge. This is the reason the legacy of Nazi science and medicine is not understood and has been largely ignored. We still have not been able to confront the time when medical science sank to its lowest depths. Nazism has become so synonymous with evil that it is invoked whenever emotions run high in ethical debates.

The Holocaust is a favourite image in protests against abortion and euthanasia, for instance. Because the Nazi analogy is so often flung around in specious ways, there has been little serious examination of those issues which legitimately do present a challenge to the ethical foundation of medicine today.

It's taken more than 40 years for modern medical science to deal with the implications of its darkest period. Why are there so few accounts of that era in bioethics journals or texts?

What ethical legacy is there in a clearly immoral chapter of history? It took a visit from Robert Pozos, a hypothermia scientist at the University of Minnesota, to convince Arthur Caplan those questions needed to be addressed.

In his work, Pozos had been citing what he thought was valuable data gathered from the cold water immersion experiments at the Dachau concentration camp. In 1942 and 1943, several hundred inmates were submerged in freezing water until death, or near death, then rewarmed, sometimes by being thrown into boiling water. This was called medical research and the doctors in charge felt it was morally justified. They were trying to find out information to help save the lives of Luftwaffe pilots whose planes were shot down over the frigid waters of the North Sea.

Unlike most data collected from concentration camp research, the Dachau data survived the war, thanks to Heinrich Himmler who buried it in a cave along with other important papers about the Third Reich. A report analysing the data was written by Leo Alexander, a major in the U.S. Army Medical Corps. The Alexander Report was used as evidence in the prosecution of Nazi war criminals. Afterwards, the document was declassified with this note on the cover page: "The Publication Board, in approving and disseminating this report, hopes that it will be of direct benefit to U.S. science and industry." The Dachau data as compiled in the report has been cited about fifty times since then in American scientific journals. Canada, Russia and Japan have also used the data in various research projects.

When Robert Pozos came to Arthur Caplan's office three years ago, he wanted to know this: is it ethical to cite the Dachau data? It was the first time anyone had bothered to ask the question. "The reason it took so long for the question to come up is that our tendency has been to push away Nazi medicine, to push away what took place in the camps, to say that was done by mad men, marginal scientists — people who could not have any relevance for what goes on in the contemporary world," says Arthur Caplan.

The myth which persists today is that only incompetent or insane doctors and scientists would willingly participate in cruel experimentation on thousands of human beings. Certainly, anyone with reputable credentials must have been coerced by the Nazi party to participate in such atrocities, and none would have felt morally or ethically justified in this behaviour.

The historical facts refute those assertions. Doctors were among the first and most numerous supporters of national socialism. 2,800 had joined the Nazi Physicians' League by early 1933 — before Hitler took power. Almost half of all

German doctors were Nazi Party members by 1943, and were heavily represented in the SS.

At the Nuremberg Doctors Trial at the end of the war, none of the 20 doctors charged with crimes against humanity pleaded insanity or said they were only following orders. In fact, these men were the cream of German medical science — leaders in their fields of research and directors of prestigious medical institutions.

All these men believed that what they did was for the benefit of society. "These were people who did not see themselves as operating in a moral vacuum; they saw themselves as operating from a strict moral code of ethics. They believed that the German nation was threatened and the threat was genetic, and that they had to do what they could to stamp it out," says Arthur Caplan who is also the editor of *When Medicine Went Mad: Bioethics and the Holocaust,* a compilation of current thought on the meaning of the Holocaust for bioethics. "Their time period was not one of moral vacuum. It was one of a jaded, twisted moral code, but it was not one in which we could say, well at least today we have values and they didn't. That is to miss the lesson. What we have today is a different set of values, a better set of values. I think we've made progress, but it's certainly the case that when one looks through the history of human experimentation in the twentieth century, one has to come to grips with the idea that evil can flow from arguments that appear to be morally sound and that are based upon ethical priniciples and language."

The operating principle of the Nazi era was eugenics — the belief that the human species could and should be improved by selective breeding. Eugenics was not a Nazi invention. The term was coined in the 1880s by British scientist Sir Francis Galton. To him and the other social Darwinists of his time, evolution was going backwards. Criminals, the disabled, the insane and the poor were growing in numbers. They threatened the survival of the better stock of people — white, middle and upper class professionals like Galton himself.

It became clear to the intellectuals in Germany that the state would have to intervene with specific policies aimed at eliminating this threat. In July 1933, the Nazi government took the first step in promoting its goal of a master race by passing "The Law for the Prevention of Genetically Diseased Offspring" — the Sterilization Law.

It was a major triumph for the German eugenics movement dedicated to the long-term care of the gene pool — called racial hygiene. Genetic health courts with doctors acting as judges recommended the sterilization of anyone they felt was defective. That included mental illness, Huntington disease, epilepsy, alcoholism and congenital blindness and deafness. By 1939, 350,000 Germans had been forcibly sterilized. It was the fulfillment of Hitler's dream as he wrote in *Mein Kampf*: "Whoever is not bodily and spiritually healthy and worthy, shall not have the right to pass on his suffering in the body of his children."

The Nazis were this century's most memorable scientific racists — but they were not the first. "There is this idea that the sterilization campaign in Nazi Germany somehow just sprang from the head of Hitler in 1933," says Angus McLaren, a professor of history at the University of Victoria and the author of *Our Own Master Race* which is the first comprehensive documentation of Canada's eugenics movement from 1885 to 1945. In fact, sterilization of the "unfit" had been widely advocated across the western world since the turn of century by respectable members of the scientific and medical communities. "It spoke to the anxieties of many people in Canada who thought that things were going wrong and of course the idea that things were going wrong in a sense peaked during the depression of the 1930s. When people were looking around to find out the causes of the nation's discomfort, it was far easier to think of these problems originating from the individual flaws of the feeble-minded, of the physically incapacitated, of the diseased, and suggest that if only these individuals were somehow removed or if they were prevented from reproducing, then the healthy people, the normal people, could get on with their lives," says McLaren.

Eugenics found most of its champions in the western provinces. In 1928, Alberta passed its own sexual sterilization act aimed at "the feeble-minded." British Columbia followed suit in 1933 — ironically the same year the Nazis came to power in Germany.

"It's interesting that the Nazis turned to Alberta. They requested the information on the Alberta legislation of 1928 to see exactly what was being done in the more progressive regions in North America," says McLaren. "There was an interchange in both directions. Canadian eugenicists thought the Nazis were brutal in many ways, in that they were perhaps crude or sometimes a little too extreme in their measures. But nevertheless, the idea was that at least the Nazis were trying to rid society of those who had to be somehow removed, who were otherwise threatening contamination for the larger community."

As in Germany, the Canadian advocates of eugenics were prominent citizens. Among its adherents were progressive women like Madge Thurlow Macklin, a leading geneticist who did important work on genetics and breast cancer. She was a fierce advocate of enforced sterilization for the mentally ill. The prestige she enjoyed as a pre-eminent scientist lent her statements a great deal of authority. The eugenics movement attracted people who have since made a name for themselves in Canadian history. For example, suffragist and future delegate to the League of Nations Nellie McClung claimed sterilization could improve morality by curbing the promiscuous behaviour of the mentally "unfit." Even CCF and NDP leader Tommy Douglas was attracted to the movement in his younger days. His M.A. thesis in sociology advocated the sterilization of criminals and prostitutes as a means to fight poverty.

In Ontario, a group of professionals founded the Eugenics Society of Canada in 1930. University professors, lawyers, public health officers and politicians joined. In 1938, the Canadian Broadcasting Corporation gave their ideas a national forum in a series of six radio addresses called "The Future of the Race." In one broadcast, the then Lieutenant-Governor of Ontario Herbert Bruce applauded Nazi Germany's efforts to deal with the problem of tainted heredity in a serious manner. He urged Canadians to do the same "biological housecleaning" and said, "It is the duty of those who direct destinies of a nation to encourage every practical means of improving the physical and mental standards of the race."

South of the border, thirty-one states eventually passed sterilization laws, beginning with Indiana in 1907, and carried out the procedure on more than

30,000 people. In 1927, the United States Supreme Court ruled that enforced sterilization was not unconstitutional. In his judgment, Justice Oliver Wendell Holmes, seen as a civil libertarian in his time, wrote: "It is better for all the world, if instead of waiting to execute degenerate offspring for crime, or to let them starve for their imbecility, society can prevent those who are manifestly unfit from continuing their kind. The principal that sustains compulsory vaccination is broad enough to cover cutting the fallopian tubes... Three generations of imbeciles are enough."

When Nazi Germany's sterilization policy turned into mass murder, the public voice favouring eugenics in North America quieted but according to Angus McLaren, there was still considerable private support for Hitler's policies. Even more remarkable is the length of time Canada's sterilization laws remained in place. "Because of the atrocities committed by the Nazis in World War Two, there was a general revulsion against eugenics. Most people assumed this type of law had disappeared. The truth is these laws were on the books until 1972," says McLaren. In Alberta, 3,000 people were sterilized. Most of them were new immigrants, natives and Metis. The records from British Columbia were lost or destroyed.

In 1939, Hitler found a more efficient way to prevent the diseased and disabled from "polluting" the gene pool of the Third Reich. A program of so-called euthanasia was in effect until 1941. It emptied the psychiatric institutions of Germany. More than 70,000 people were killed in hospital gas chambers. This was the rehearsal for the "Final Solution." The doctors and the gas chambers were moved to Poland — the Nazis called this "the great therapy of Auschwitz." For William Seidelman, this descent down the slippery slope is what we must remember. "The scientific rationalization for the wholesale destruction of human life occurred in medicine. The gas chamber and crematoria that we associate with death camps originated in German psychiatric hospitals. The first victims were patients in these hospitals. When that program of so-called euthanasia ended, the personnel and the equipment were shipped to the death camps. It originated in medicine and was part of the mainstream and many people involved in that program were in fact professors of medicine."

What is also striking about the Nazi "euthanasia" program is the way in which the general public was convinced to go along with it.

When Nazi Germany chose killing people as the way to rid society of contaminants, its propaganda machine went into overdrive. Films portraying people with disabilities and mental illness as evil flickered on movie screens all over the country. They were the highlight of the campaign to sell mass murder to the German public. "In 1939 there were dozens of films with titles like 'Genetic Disease' and 'Genetic Threat' and 'The Menace of the Disabled'. They whipped up a kind of fear and hatred. Parents were made to feel horror at having a malformed child or disabled relative. Then of course the question of voluntary is lost as well. Basically people are informed that because of a genetic impairment or mental handicap they are going to be forcibly relieved of their suffering," says Robert Proctor, associate professor of history at Pennsylvania State University and the author of *Racial Hygiene: Medicine Under the Nazis*.

The catch phrase of the Nazi "euthanasia" program was "lives not worth living." Economic arguments were used to reinforce racial hygiene policies. Spending scarce health care resources on so-called "useless eaters" did not make sense. "They believed that sacrificing the few for the interests of the many was appropriate. They believed that if the state were burdened by costly groups — the mentally ill, the retarded, the elderly — then doctors had a role to play in containing those costs. And if that meant letting those people die or committing active euthanasia upon them, then that's what the doctor ought to do," says Arthur Caplan.

We cannot easily dismiss half a century of modern scientific thinking as an aberration or an unfortunate by-product of a vile and racist ideology. It is arrogant and naive to cling to the belief that all that is behind us, argues Robert Proctor. "You'll often read in scientific journals that doctors or scientists were just victims of the Nazi presence, but in fact they were willing supporters. And if scientists then could have become so easily entranced with Nazi priorities, how are things different today? I think that's one of the questions we have to ask. Scientists are susceptible to the social forces of their time and they are more often ethical followers than leaders, I would say. And if that's true, then whatever social problems we have are liable to be reflected in the structure of the science we do. So, I'm very wary of admitting that we've learned properly our lesson from the Nazi period."

The Nazi goal of purifying the biology of the population was designed by the world's greatest scientific minds. Germany was the birthplace of modern medical science and the model for the university-based medical school. "The fact remains that Germany, during the twentieth century and up until the time of World War Two, was probably the premier biomedical and scientific nation on the face of the earth," says Arthur Caplan, "and if they could find themselves experimenting on children or prisoners of war or Jews or Gypsies in camps, I think it's hard for us to ask the question because it makes us look deep within ourselves and wonder if we could be capable of the same thing. And it's something we don't want to ask."

The lesson is not about evil doctors. It's not about how the Nazis corrupted science and medicine but the fact that distinguished members of the scientific and medical community engineered policies of scientific racism. "It is essentially a story about power and abuse of that power. What I feel the medical profession and the health professions have to consider is the question of the physician as a human being, as a vulnerable, fallible person who makes mistakes. And I think it's important to look at this particular tragic epoch as an example of the vulnerability of the profession," says William Seidelman.

No area of biomedical science draws more analogies to the Nazi era than genetics. Arthur Caplan believes there is a crucial link: "The most relevant fact is that we have to deal with history when we look at genetics. It's not a question of could we abuse things, or might dangerous or evil things happen. They did. Genetics is an area where we know that sophisticated, intelligent, capable and competent scientists and doctors could do genocide in the name of biology."

With the birth of molecular biology after the war came the ability to identify specific genes. Crude eugenic arguments about selective breeding were dismissed and replaced with a more sophisticated and somehow less sinister terminology and science. We are now exploring a scientific frontier eugenicists and Nazi doctors could only dream of.

Scientists all over the world are now trying to isolate and identify the 50,000-100,000 genes in the human body. This international effort is called the Human Genome Organization. For its part, the United States is spending three billion dollars over fifteen years on efforts to map and sequence the human genome. About five percent of the budget has been set aside to study the ethics of using the findings.

The U.S. Human Genome Project has excited the genetics community and captured the imagination of the general public. The hope is that once we know what certain genes do, we will know much more about what causes diseases and how to cure them. But at the same time there are worries that this new information is not going to be value-free. If we reduce ourselves to a human bar code, how will science and society define what is "normal" or "abnormal?"

For now, the proponents of the U.S. Human Genome Project maintain that we are smart enough to avoid that trap. "This time around we do have the past to guide us. That is, we've seen the dangers of trying to establish a particular version of the human form and psyche as a model and trying to force the rest of the population into it," says Eric Juengst, the director of the Ethical, Legal and Social Implications program of the Human Genome Project. "That was the old-style eugenics movement of the '30s and '40s. And it's not something I think our society would go back to very easily, or should go back to."

But Robert Proctor, who has received a grant from the project's ethics budget, feels that's easier said than done. "One of the slogans of the Nazi period was 'national socialism is just applied biology'. They might as well have said applied genetics. I think the notion of biology as destiny is getting stronger again."

Proctor is one of a growing number of critics who feel that the promise of the new genetic technology is creating a blind spot to the pitfalls. "When Nazi racial biology or racial hygiene was discredited after World War Two, there was a strong resurgence of environmentalist theories and people argued for the importance of education and potentiality. But much of that has lapsed again. I think it's a kind of memory phenomenon. Enough time has passed that few people remember World War Two and much of its legacy. I think that's one of the reasons we're getting a resurgence in biological determinism."

American frustration about escalating inner-city crime had the Bush administration looking to our genes for answers. A controversial research program on violence launched by the U.S. National Institute of Mental Health last year included a plan to find genetic markers for criminal behaviour in young black children. The U.S. government's acceptance of the idea that genetic deficiencies could cause social problems was demonstrated again in the fall of 1992. The National Institutes of Health were prepared to fund a conference called "Genetic Factors in Crime: Findings, Uses and Implications." The brochure advertising the three day conference to be held at the University of Maryland read: "Genetic research holds out the prospect of identifying individuals who may be predisposed to certain kinds of criminal conduct." Vigorous protests put the conference on hold. In March 1993, it was finally cancelled.

But it left many people including Robert Proctor fearing that scientific racism is regaining legitimacy in mainstream science. "I think it's an incredibly dangerous and disturbing fact that so many biologists are willing to entertain the idea that crime might be genetic. The Nazis were pioneers on this and effectively argued that certain racial groups were not only disposed to crime, but disposed to particular types of crime. So the Nazis talked about the Gypsies being shiftless and natural thieves, genetic thieves; the Jews being genetically oriented toward financial crime. I think it shows people are grasping for straws in trying to explain away crime," says Proctor.

The resurgence of the notion of biology as destiny is best exemplified in the work of Canadian researcher Philippe Rushton. He is a psychology professor at the University of Western Ontario who has been conducting a project to assess racial differences in intelligence, brain size, sex drive control and lawfulness. He has concluded that Blacks rank at the bottom, Caucasians are on the next rung, with Asians at the top.

Rushton's work and in fact much of the research into inherited intelligence conducted in North America and Western Europe is sponsored by the Pioneer Fund, a small, private New York-based group. It was founded in 1937 by millionaire alumni of Harvard and Princeton who had a keen interest in eugenics. The most involved research supported by the Pioneer Fund is the Minnesota Study of Twins Reared Apart headed by Thomas Bouchard Jr. For more than a dozen years Bouchard's team has been studying more than one hundred sets of identical and fraternal twins who grew up in separate environments. In 1990, Bouchard published his conclusion: "Seventy percent of the variance in IQ was found to be associated with genetic variation." This was incorrectly taken to mean that seventy percent of IQ was due to genes.

Because the Pioneer Fund sponsors projects which favour genes over environment as a determinant of intelligence, critics label it a supporter of race science and an organization that is still firmly rooted in eugenic ideals. Those charges are worrisome considering there are few hereditary research projects which do not receive some money from the Pioneer Fund.

As well, there has been a renewed interest in brain differences between heterosexuals and homosexuals. And with each new discovery of a gene linked to a specific disorder or disease, our fascination is piqued even more. "One of the most bizarre ones I saw recently was a study that argued that couch potatoism was partially genetic and that people watched different types of TV shows according to their genetic propensity. I told this to a colleague who started nodding and said, yeah, maybe there is something to that," says Proctor who feels it is the sheer simplicity of genetic explanations makes them so attractive. "It's very seductive. If you can say it's all in our genes — the problem is at root a biological one — it's a soothing kind of notion. I think it's something very similar to the old line that if you got a severe disease it was the hand of God. Now you can simply say it's the working out of genetic determinism."

One day there might be hundreds, even thousands of genetic tests which can identify diseases and traits of all kinds. But what are we going to do with the information and what will we do to the people who carry these genes? Two recent Canadian reports on genetics offer very different perspectives.

A 1991 Science Council of Canada report called *Genetics in Canadian Health Care* paints a rosy picture of advances in genetic technology which are "used in a way that maximizes their benefits and minimizes any potential harm." Dr. Charles Scriver is the report's author and a geneticist at the Montreal Children's Hospital and McGill University's Human Genetics Centre. "There's no eugenic option in this. Eugenics is a population policy that says it knows what's good for you or what's bad for you. What we are talking about is providing components in a health care system that will allow people to have tests and make choices," says Scriver, adding that critics of genetics testing are fearful of change. "A lot of people objected to the pasteurization of milk. They said that this was contaminating one of God's most important foods. Do you really believe this was a bad decision? We're saying genetics and health care is rather like fifty years ago, having X-ray machines in hospitals. Can you imagine the Canadian health care system without diagnostic imaging today? No."

In the report's section on ethics, the chances for potential harm are minimized: "The 'slippery slope' argument is often raised against the use of genetic technologies. The implication is that once initial steps are taken, there is no recognizable appropriate place to stop the use of genetic technology. The argument does not hold. Responsible distinctions can be made between a therapeutic application of a genetic technology, a trivial use, and the implementation of population eugenics. Moral decisions regarding the use of genetic technologies can and should be made by individuals and society."

The Science Council report argues that the objective of genetic testing is to give families the freedom to make informed choices. "Medical geneticists in Canada today are clearly oriented to individual and family needs and are not primarily concerned with the impact of parental reproductive choice on society, let alone the human species." The report goes on to assure us that medical geneticists in Canada and elsewhere in the world can rightfully reject any link between their work and the eugenics policies of the 1930s and '40s.

The thrust of a 1992 report from the office of the Privacy Commissioner of Canada called *Genetic Testing and Privacy* adopts quite another tone: "One is struck by the parallel between unlocking the gene in the '90s and unlocking the atom in the '40s. In both cases the excitement of the discovery dulled critical assessment of the implications. In both cases we allowed scientists to unleash forces which can alter life as we know it, paid for their efforts with public funds and, at least initially, set few ethical or legal controls on the enterprises."

This report emphasizes that genetic technology has the capacity to reveal the most intimate secrets about ourselves and it will take more than a sense of decency and civility to prevent others from exploiting that information or even protect the right not to know our own genetic destiny. "The threat to privacy is but one of a host of possible genetic 'evils' that must be countered now before we are trampled by the march of the technology," warns the report.

The Human Genome Organization is the most ambitious endeavour of its kind in history. It has been heralded as everything from "the new biology" to "the Quest for the Holy Grail." The U.S. Project's first director was James Watson, who is still remembered for this statement on the potential benefits for the human race: "How can we not do it? We used to think that our fate is in our stars. Now we know, in large measure, our fate is in our genes."

It is language like that which makes genomics look like a sacred quest, something that only good can come from. It tends to discourage very deep thinking, argues George Annas, a professor of health law at Boston University and the author of *Gene Mapping: Using Law and Ethics as Guides*. "We've heard this all before, that it's just a matter of accustoming ourselves to the technology," says Annas. "It's naïve to think that a project that is going to make us capable of identifying differences in individuals at the molecular level is not going to lead to discriminating against people based on their genomes. It's time we should start learning some lessons from history and be a little more suspicious about people who tell us that knowledge of genetics is going to make the world better, and make us all able to live together better, when history teaches us that knowledge of genetic differences usually makes things a lot worse."

It's not necessary to go back sixty years to find an example of the dark side of what we can do with a little genetic knowledge. "In the 1970s sickle cell anemia screening was being used to identify those people who had either sickle cell anemia or sickle cell trait," recounts Eugene Oscapella, an Ottawa lawyer and author of *Genetic Testing and Privacy.* "Now most of the people who have that trait happen to be black. So if you find someone with sickle cell anemia, chances are that person is black and of course if you want to discriminate on the basis of race, that's a very convenient way of doing it. You just say, well, we don't want to hire you because you've got sickle cell anemia, when in fact it may be used as a tool for discriminating on the basis of race. Basically, if you can identify information about people, you can use that information to discriminate against them."

Insurance companies are already exploiting genetic information. A pregnant American woman was told she would lose her family's health coverage if she gave birth to her baby because prenatal testing revealed that her unborn child had cystic fibrosis. Another woman who had a fifty-fifty chance of developing Huntington disease had her life insurance revoked. Our view of what is a disease, a disability or an enhancement may change over time. There have been cases of parents asking their doctors for genetically engineered human growth hormone to make their children taller. Is shortness now an impairment? It is fine to say there are tremendous potential benefits arising from the technology and we need to make sure the information is used in a responsible manner. But in a debate where ethics are relegated to the realm of benefits, critics' voices tend to be marginalized.

The technology is on a fast track to tell us a child's genetic makeup before it is born. Prenatal testing is the most common application of genetic technology in humans today. Women over the age of 35 are routinely offered tests for Down syndrome and spina bifida through amniocentesis, chorionic villus sampling or new maternal blood tests which indicate risk factors for those hereditary diseases. The line between preventing the birth of fetuses with severe defects and improving the species begins to blur.

And who decides which prenatal tests should be developed? Why have we spent so much time and money looking for fetuses with Down syndrome? At what point are we dealing with the concept of designing a "better" human being? These are questions being asked by watchdog groups such as the Boston-based Council for Responsible Genetics. It would like to see some answers before more and more tests are added.

The lines between the fit and unfit are being drawn in today's laboratories. Advocates for the disabled are also worried about where these value judgments are leading. "We're now witnessing the development of the technology to prevent people from being born by detecting that they will have a disability before birth, and to encourage the mother to have an abortion," says Orville Endicott, legal council to the Canadian Association for Community Living in Toronto. "Now that illustrates the focus that society and particularly professional medicine has developed. Let's make sure that these people aren't born. They ought not to be born. And of course that says a great deal about those who have already been born and are likely to be treated as people who ought not to have been born. And when it comes to society's health care resources, that will be in people's minds."

In a real sense we are determining who our "useless eaters" are. Germany felt it was spending scarce resources feeding and caring for people who had no value to society. In the past, eugenic goals were achieved through social policy, sterilization and murder. Today, our knowledge of molecular biology means we have real power to impose our genetic ideals before birth.

George Annas puts it this way. Two visions of western society's future emerged after World War Two — both embodied in literature. In *1984* George Orwell saw totalitarian governments taking over the world ruthlessly forcing their ideologies on people. In Aldous Huxley's "Brave New World," there would be no need for the controlling force of "Big Brother." Governments would be able to manipulate citizens through mass media and drugs like "soma" into wanting to do what the state demanded. Annas feels Huxley's view of our destiny is much more likely. We like new knowledge and new medicine. If we believe that the application of genetic technology will help us lead more fulfilled lives, then we will demand it.

There are powerful forces at work in our society that could create a culture where people are judged by their genetic endowments, argues Annas. "Probably most couples will want to know any information that could help them have a healthier baby, or a baby that has a better chance to compete in the world. So I think we don't need governments forcing people to use the new genetic information with regard to human reproduction. I think people want to do that."

According to Annas the driving forces of eugenics already make up the fabric of western society — our quest for immortality, our pursuit of progress which leads to a more perfect world, and damn the consequences. "The dream is that someday we'll be able to treat all these genetic diseases. In fact, we haven't found the first one that we can treat yet. For at least the foreseeable future, mostly we'll be identifying things we can't do anything about, except worry."

The field of biomedical ethics is trying to come to terms with our eugenic past to prevent similar mistakes in applying our new genetic knowledge. There are scientists and physicians who feel such an effort is irrelevant, even impertinent. Their attitude toward ethical considerations is one of convenience. If ethics can be co-opted to support their research agendas, it is worth considering. But whenever ethicists caution us about the potential dangers of science, their concerns are dismissed as "fear of the unknown."

Arthur Caplan, among many others, believes this thinking misses the point. He subscribes to the well-known thesis of philosopher George Santayana who said that those who ignore the past are condemned to repeat it. "When people try to justify the research today by saying it would be good for the state or good for the general public health, that it would justify sacrificing the vulnerable or the few or the incompetent, we've got to keep our ears up because that's exactly how the Nazis wound up where they did."

For Eva Mozes-Kor, who along with her twin sister Miriam survived a year-long ordeal in Dr. Mengele's laboratory at Auschwitz, the last frontier in the landscape of today's scientific debate may be our own morality. "If they are doing any research, they are doing it for the sake of humanity. The moment they forget that they are not only doctors and scientists, but human beings dealing with human beings, they are very much approaching the arrogance of Mengele."

BIBLIOGRAPHY

Annas, George and Elias, Sherman (eds.), *Gene Mapping: Using Law and Ethics as Guides*, Oxford University Press, 1992.

Annas, George and Grodin, Michael (eds.), *The Nazi Doctors and Nuremberg Code: Human Rights in Human Experimentation*, Oxford University Press, 1992.

Caplan, Arthur (ed.), *When Medicine Went Mad: Bioethics and the Holocaust*, Humana Press, 1992.

Kater, Michael H., *Doctors Under Hitler*, University of North Carolina Press, 1989.

Lifton, Robert Jay, *The Nazi Doctors: Medical Killing and the Psychology of Genocide*, Basic Books, 1986.

McLaren, Angus, *Our Own Master Race: Eugenics in Canada, 1885-1945*, McClelland & Stewart, 1990.

[The] Privacy Commissioner of Canada, *Genetic Testing and Privacy* 1992.

Proctor, Robert, *Racial Hygiene: Medicine Under the Nazis*, Harvard University Press, 1988.

[The] Science Council of Canada, *Genetics In Canadian Health Care, 1991*.

6

FROM COW SHED TO CLINIC: VETERINARY SCIENCE AND THE NEW REPRODUCTIVE AND GENETIC TECHNOLOGIES

Annette Burfoot

Over the past 10 to 15 years, the assisted RTs [reproductive technologies] have revolutionized the treatment of human infertility... including [the] male factor... and created opportunities for the preservation of endangered non-human species and for the development of improved disease models for medical research.[1]

It is important to understand the recent developments in human reproductive technologies in context of the science of all reproduction (including genetics) and commercial applications of this understanding (particularly in the areas of veterinary science and animal husbandry). *In vitro* fertilization (IVF) acts as the central component of these relationships and is related to the three main areas: veterinary science and animal husbandry; medical practice and genetic engineering. These three areas are also directly related to each other, sometimes in the same time period and sometimes over time. The entire system is related to commercial interests since, at each moment in time and in each of the areas financial success has played an important role. What follows is an explanation of the inter-relationships between IVF, and veterinary science and animal husbandry.

VETERINARIAN SCIENCE AND ANIMAL HUSBANDRY

The line between non-human animal research and human research has never been clear and, as we will see shortly, interactions between the two move in both directions. For example, we often use non-human animals in research and tests for human's benefit (in matters of reproduction). Many of the current advanced techniques used in human reproduction come from experimentation on non-human animals and applications in the agricultural industries. But as Professor John Hearn, former head of the MRC/AFRC Comparative Physiology Research Group at London's Institute of Zoology (The London Zoo), explains, IVF also reverses this trend in that animal specialists turn to human work in IVF for explanations of non-human reproduction and embryology as most IVF now takes place with humans[2]. Zoologists use IVF to propagate endangered species as non-domesticated animals are often unlikely to reproduce in captivity.

In Australia, a record price of $300,000 (US) was paid for a merino ram to provide semen to be used in breeding.[3] The high price for the ram was attributed to new breeding techniques taken from recent human applications, including IVF, embryo freezing and embryo transfer, which enable the creature to produce more genetic offspring than through "conventional" approaches. Also, the physiological similarities between humans and other animals encourages collaborative and combination research; it is very common to find embryologists trained for agricultural research and commercial breeding firms working in newly established IVF clinics.

Hearn admits that many of the technicians his unit has trained in non-human embryology have gone to IVF clinics. In the University of Vermont's Medical Centre, where a small IVF practice was established in 1985, an embryologist from the nearby agricultural college (Vermont is a large dairy producer) was originally responsible for the lab work required in the IVF unit as well as for training new technicians in human IVF lab procedures.[4] It is common for embryologists whose specialities are non-human species to work in conjunction with human IVF applications. At times, these specialists apply their expertise in the human context and at other times they participate in the procedures for their own research purposes.

HISTORY OF NEW REPRODUCTIVE TECHNOLOGIES

Typically, the history of IVF and related techniques has moved in the opposite direction: from non-human to human. K.J. Betteridge has researched extensively the history of embryo transfer in non-human animals[5] and makes clear the veterinary precedent for IVF as a medical practice. An illustration of this follows.

Walter Heape, a nineteenth century biologist and pioneer in embryo transfer, was recently featured in a centenary celebration of the technique.[6] Heape was the first to successfully transfer rabbit embryos from the genetic mother to a recipient. It appears that the term "success" did not mean a live birth but the establishment of a pregnancy in the host. Most of the early transferred embryos were lost soon after implantation — it was not until 1951 when the synchronization of hormones in the recipient and the donor were fully appreciated that the first transferred mammal (a calf) was born. Further evidence of the interconnected nature of non-human and human reproductive engineering is that the 100 year anniversary of embryo transfer (used initially and widely in animal husbandry for breeding livestock) is celebrated in a journal dealing with human reproduction.

Heape, and those scientists like him, inadvertently caused increased interest in human reproduction by splitting it from birth (a low status medical preoccupation) and making it worthy of scientific investigation into unchartered biotechnological territory. They also engaged with a growing industry in livestock with new capabilities to manage and maximize breeding. Science had become linked with commerce (in this case agriculture) and a profit motive.

ARTIFICIAL INSEMMINATION

In the early twentieth century artificial insemination was already in use by livestock breeders. As Betteridge notes, artificial insemination (AI) — reportedly used widely by the Russians in livestock breeding since the 1930s — was an important step towards successful embryo implantation as both a precedent for managed conception and a source of new information drawn from the experience of AI such as sperm preparation, storage and handling. In 1926, British sheep semen was being delivered through the mail to farms throughout Britain, continental Europe and America. This demonstrates how AI was appreciated by the farming and agricultural industries as useful in quickly disseminating desired genetic traits and maximizing the production capabilities of livestock.

As the international demand for donor semen rose, freezing techniques were developed to cope with storage and transport problems. Chris Polge, with his Cambridge colleagues in 1949, discovered how to freeze sperm without damaging it. More recently, scientists have developed a glycerol-based cryopreservation medium for sustaining frozen human embryos.

There was very little hesitation in making the transition from artificial insemination (the transfer of semen) to embryo transfer in livestock. The difference between the two procedures is that with embryo transfer, desirable genetic traits of females as well as males could be transferred widely, whereas semen transfer could only transfer male genetic traits. By 1949, a farming and research unit in San Antonio, Texas had attempted embryo transfer in 750 cows over a seven-year period in anticipation of the commercial prospects for transporting embryos with the desired genetic contributions from both parents. Although none of these transplants were successful in terms of live births, the attempts raised sufficient international interest to justify the first conference devoted to embryo transfer in San Antonio in 1949. The first live birth of a calf as a result of embryo transfer occurred in Wisconsin (1951) at another large livestock research centre. Today, Betteridge reports that it is not unusual for a single commercial embryo-transfer firm to complete 3,000 transfers a year and there is an international trade in embryos for stock breeding purposes.[7]

Traditionally, eggs for embryo transfer were removed from female livestock in the slaughter house although surgical techniques were developed earlier. The eggs of slaughtered animals were easily accessible, cheap, sufficient for research and also suitable for providing embryos for donation. Obviously, this procedure was inadequate when the animal was alive and its breeders wanted to keep her that way as a future resource for breeding. Similarly, women's ovaries were often taken after sterilization procedures for experimentation — this is how Robert Edwards, one of the first to succeed with the IVF technique in humans, started his research. Because, both the cows and the women were valued alive with their reproductive capacities intact, more refined surgical techniques were developed as early as 1928 so that eggs could be removed from live women's (and cows') fallopian tubes. In 1955 the process of flushing embryos from sheep was developed.[9]

The possibility of embryo transfer started with scientific interest in the nature of reproduction and was consequently fueled by the commercial potential of the technique as applied to livestock breeding. Yet throughout its development, the human application of embryo transfer for scientific and clinical purposes was never forgotten. Heape's early experiments with rabbits were designed to increase understanding of the process of reproduction in all mammals, including women. In the late nineteenth century, hardly anything was known of the role of hormones in reproduction and much was speculated about the roles of the fallopian tubes and uterus in conception. Scientific knowledge has not developed much further in this regard. Some early culture mediums used for IVF contained ground tissues from the uterus and fallopian tubes in the presumption that some essence was contained there that would promote fertilization. This hypothesis has since been abandoned and a new one has been established which deals with the bio-chemicals involved in natural conception, particularly sugars.

Besides the early work of the nineteenth century biologists, there was research at Yale where rat viability tests in 1933 established the importance of hormonal synchronicity between donor and the rats. Work on sheep and goat hybrids was performed in Texas in 1934; the researchers there were interested in the function of the uterine environment as a possible deterrent to breeding hybrids. In 1935, cancer research in mice required embryo transfer techniques. Wisconsin was testing the viability of cow embryos produced with superovulation in 1944 and in 1951 Edinburgh scientists used embryo transfer in mice during their research in genetics. Robert Edwards (who along with Patrick Steptoe, directed the first successful "test-tube baby" experiment) completed his Ph.D. in mouse genetics at the University of Edinburgh in the mid-1950's.

RECENT DEVELOPMENTS

This trend in reproductive engineering continues today with the control of disease in pre-implantation cow and pig embryos[10] and genetic manipulation. Techniques now used in beef and dairy production include nucleus breeding (the micromanipulation of reproductive cells), cloning (asexual reproduction used to enhance desired genetic traits) and twinning (splitting eggs prior to IVF and implantation to produce twins).[11] Also, AIDS researchers are now interested in bovine immunodeficiency virus (BIV) as it mimics the AIDS virus.

The most recent discoveries and applications in non-human reproduction are likely to have an impact on human research and clinical applications. It is this very link that many countries identify and attempt to break in their recommendations for legislation that bans cross-species fertilization and cloning with human gametes.[12] Research that does not involve human gametes is permitted, however, in order to "improve" livestock and to investigate possibilities in human reproduction.[13]

The more recent veterinarian and animal husbandry developments in this regard include the following: Sheep tetraparental chimeras (the genetic recombination of same-species but different types) were created in the early 1970s[14] shortly followed by the sexing of cow blastocysts *in vitro* prior to implantation[15] and the creation of identical twins in sheep by splitting the embryo at a very early stage of its development.[16] Now inter-species chimeras are possible. For example, in 1984 the "geep" emerged from crossing a sheep with a goat, again using the micromanipulation of eggs and sperm. There have also been "ligers" and "tigrons" as well as animals fortified with genetic information from other species.

Micromanipulation of gametes and embryos is used in the same way but in different contexts in humans and non-human species for improving conception rates. In humans, micromanipulation, in conjunction with IVF, is used to diagnose and counter male infertility while in experimental zoology, it assists with the preservation of endangered species.[17] Pre-implantation embryo sexing is experimented with in both humans and non-human species. In cattle, it is applied in the dairy industry to create a majority of cows (and a minimum of bulls) for maximizing milk potentials.[18] In humans, it is used for eugenic purposes (desired genetic outcome such as the sex of the child). Alternative gestation sites are also being explored in non-human species: Mouse embryos are implanted just under the skin of mouse hosts.[19]

CONCLUSIONS

There are a host of questions and problems that arise from the interconnections between new reproductive technologies, the animal industry and veterinary science. Because IVF is a new procedure, which depends heavily on science for its application and further development, a new convergence occurs between medical practitioners and scientific researchers (particularly from human and non-human reproductive physiology and genetics). This co-operation creates unique funding situations for IVF as it is simultaneously a clinical practice and a trials site, a research program and a site for commercial applications. Direct commercial interests underwrite the cost of pure research and provide clinical training while public bodies fund the medical practice and also support related scientific research. As such, it is difficult to determine the exact amount of public funds going to new reproductive technologies and commercial motivations are hard to separate from scientific and medical concerns.

Technological capabilities developed in non-human animals are often determined outside of the scope of medical ethics. As such, agendas for the breeding of animals for human consumption, for example, may design reproductive technologies that are eventually applied to women. This practice also serves as an experimental site not only for human reproductive techniques but also for pure research in veterinary reproductive science. Finally, the high status and potential profit of genetic engineering lends further rationale for the continuance of IVF and related procedures and places greater emphasis on genetic continuity and eugenics (the science of improving the population by control of inherited qualities). In this environment of heightened interest in and practice of eugenic breeding in livestock and race horses, there is a concurrent and related trend towards eugenics in human reproduction (i.e., sex selection of pre-implantation embryos).

Other possible technological transfers to human application could be the routinization of testing of women's pregnancies and pre-implantion embryos for a variety of genetic-linked diseases and viruses (such as HIV). Doctors have proposed that pre-implantation diagnosiscould become routine practice in IVF programs. Such techniques are already applied to control undesired genetic outcomes and viruses in livestock herds and race horses. Nucleus breeding schemes also enhance eugenic programs in animal breeding and could be applied to humans for genetic engineering purposes as well as for basic science research on embryos for the purposes of furthering knowledge about human development. As experimental sites for the science of reproduction (including the diagnosis and treatment of male infertility) women are becoming the animal models for breeding techniques which are not restricted to human use. This further obscures women's humanity with the motives and requirements of a research agenda closely tied historically and economically with the animal breeding industry and veterinary science.

NOTES

1   Don Wolf, (ed.) *Seminars in Reproductive Endocrinology: Assisted Reproductive Technologies and Male Infertility.* vol. 11, no. 1, February 1993.

2   Interview with John Hearn, London, August 14, 1987 and September 2, 1988.

3   "Australia: Record Price for Merino Ram," *Financial Times.* October 10, 1988, p.42.

4   Interview with Paul Riddick, Department of Obstetrics and Gynaecology, Mary Fletcher Hospital, Burlington, Vermont, USA., January 19, 1987.

5   K.J. Betteridge, "An Historical Look at Embryo Transfer," *Journal of Reproduction and Fertility.* vol. 62, 1981.

6   J.D. Biggers, "Walter Heape, FRS: A Pioneer in Reproductive Biology. Centenary of His Embryo Transfer Experiments," *The Journal of Reproduction and Fertility.* vol. 93, September 1991, pp. 173-86.

7   "Animal Breeding Company has World-Wide Experience of Embryo Transfer," *Agriculture International.* vol. 40, February 1988, p. s13.

8   E. Allen, J.P. Pratt, Q.U. Newell and L. Bland, "Recovery of Human Ova from the Uterine Tubes: Time of Ovulation in the Menstrual Cycles," *The Journal of the American Medical Association.* vol. 91 (1928) pp. 1018-1020.

9 G.L. Hunter, C.E. Adams and L.E.A Rowson, "Interbreed Ovum Transfer in Sheep," *Journal of Agricultural Science.* vol. 46 (1955) p.143.

10 R.F. DiGiacomo, et al, "Failure of Embryo Transfer to Transmit BLV in a Dairy Herd," *The Veterinary Record.* vol. 127, November 3, 1990, p.456;

J. E. James, et al, "Embryo Transfer for Conserving Valuable Genetic Material from Swine Herds with Pseudorabies," *Journal of the American Veterinary Medical Association.* vol. 183, September 1983, pp. 525-8.

11 George Teepker, and David S. Keller, "Selection of Sires Originating from a Nucleus Breeding Unit for Use in a Commercial Dairy Population," *Canadian Journal of Animal Science.* vol. 69, September 1989, pp. 595-604;

C. Smith, "Cloning and Genetic Improvement of Beef Cattle," *Animal Production.* vol. 49, August 1989, pp. 49-62;

J.A. Wooliams, "Modifications to MOET Nucleus Breeding Schemes to Improve Rates of Genetic Progress...," *Animal Production.* vol. 49, August 1989, pp. 1-14;

J.A. Wooliams, "The Value of Cloning in MOET Nucleus Breeding Schemes for Dairy Cattle," *Animal Production.* vol. 48, February 1989, pp. 31-5.

12 For example, the British legislation on new reproductive technologies prohibits trans-species procreation with humans.

13 R.B. Heap, et al, "Oestrogen Production by the Implantation Donkey Conceptus Compared with that of the Horse and the Effect of Between-Species Embryo Transfer," *Journal of Reproduction and Fertility.* vol. 93, September 1991, pp. 141-7;

Duane C. Kraemer, "Intra- and Interspecific Embryo Transfer," *The Journal of Experimental Zoology.* vol. 228, November 1983, pp. 203-13.

14 E.M. Tucker, R.M. Moor, L.E.A. Rowson, "Tetraparental Sheep Chimeras Induced by Blastomere Transplantation," *Immunology.* vol. 26 (1974) pp. 613-621.

15 W.C.D. Hare, D. Mitchell, K.J. Betteridge, M.D. Eaglesome and G.C.B. Randall, "Sexing Two Week-old Bovine Embryos by Chromosomal Analysis Prior to Surgical Transfer," *Pheriogeneology.* vol.5 (1976) pp.243-253.

16 "A Method for Culture of Micro-manipulated Sheep Embryos and its use to Produce Monozygotic Twins," *Nature.* vol. 227 (1979) pp. 298-300.

17 Mina Alikani, and Cohen Jacques, "Micromanipulation of Cleaved Embryos cultured in Protein-Free Medium: A Mouse Model for Assisted Hatching," *The Journal of Experimental Zoology.* vol. 263, October 1, 1992, pp. 458-63.

18 Colleau, J. J., "Using Embryo Sexing Within Closed Mixed Multiple Ovulation and Embryo Transfer Schemes for Selection on Dairy Cattle," *Journal of Dairy Science.* vol. 74, November 1991, pp. 3973-84.

19 Bevilacqua, Estela Marvis A. F. and Paulo A. Abrahamson, "Growth of Mouse Embryos Implanted in the Subcutaneous Tissue of Recipient Mice," *The Journal of Experimental Zoology.* vol. 257, March 1991, pp. 386-400.

7

HOW OLD MCDONALD LOST THE FARM AND DOCTORS GOT TO 'MAKE' BABIES: A PERSONAL REFLECTION ON THE REPRODUCTIVE INDUSTRY

Gwynne Basen

Science Finds — Industry Applies — Man Conforms

Motto of 1933 World's Fair

A cow is being led into a holding pen at Alta Genetics Inc. The Alberta company is one of the leaders in high-tech cattle breeding. Heavy metal bars are put up around the cow. They make a fearsome clanging sound that reverberates off the cement floors and walls. The bars are pulled in tighter until the cow cannot possibly move. This cow has been here before and no longer tries to resist.

The technician's arm is covered in a rubber glove that goes past his elbow. He sticks his hand deep into the cow's rectum. Her large brown eyes open wider but she doesn't make a sound. Another man sets up a long plastic tube that goes into her uterus. Pink liquid from a bottle attached above flows into her and out again, flushing the embryos from her womb. When they are finished another cow is led in. The bars go up around her. The technician wheels over an ultrasound machine. He sticks the probe into her rectum and an image appears on the small screen. This cow is pregnant and the buyer wants information on the product — is the fetus male or female? — before he'll close the sale.

In the IVF clinic at the University Hospital in London, Ontario, a doctor inserts a vaginal probe between the bent legs of the woman lying on the table. She is covered by a white sheet. The doctor talks to her as he looks at the black and white shapes on the ultrasound screen. "O.K. Kathy, this is your uterus. It's a nice uterus." The doctor is looking for ripe follicles.

Those two scenes follow one another in a film called *Making Babies*. It is the first of two films on the reproductive and genetic technologies I directed in 1992.[1] That cut, from the barn to the clinic, from the cow to the woman, makes a lot of women angry. It should, that's one of the reasons we did it. Only sometimes they get angry at me! In confusing the message with the messenger, I have been accused of "equating women with research animals," and "repeatedly comparing women with cattle."[2] I didn't go looking for cows, they were there. The comparisons, the equations, were everywhere. I didn't create them. I just observed them, thought about them, and in the end, put some in the film.

We can't ignore what goes on in those barns. Most of the reproductive and genetic technologies now in use have come to the clinics from the barn yard. It's there I saw new techniques that will soon become part of human reproductive experimentation. Technology has already irrevocably changed human procreation. And if we do nothing to stop it, that transformation will continue until making babies becomes another industrial process, becomes (re)production.

* * * * *

A bull floats above the earth in a starry sky. The words across the top of the brochure read, "Protein and Profit. Meeting the demand for high protein genetics world wide." The goals of the cattle breeding industry are very clear. "Precision genetics. Personalized service," reads the glossy colour brochure of United Breeders in Guelph, Ontario. The man I speak with there tells me that producing these booklets is their single major expenditure. On the inside pages are the "beauty" shots. Cows groomed to perfection and carefully arranged to show off their best features: pendulous and productive udders. Underneath are their stats, proof that these cows have what it takes. "Canadian genetics are a solid investment."

Every technological development in the cattle industry has one aim: to improve productivity and increase profits. "An embryonic market bonanza," is the headline of a 1980 *Maclean's* Magazine piece about embryo freezing. "If successful, the technique could revolutionize the cattle breeding industry..."

Current shipping costs are "almost $900 an animal, decreasing its competitiveness in the world market.... The idea of being able to carry a whole herd in a suitcase is fantastic." The two scientists involved in embryo freezing reported a success rate of 33 percent — "We've got lots of work to do yet."

Six months later an Australian newspaper reported that doctors in that country had been freezing human embryos for over a year: "Babes on Ice in Test Tube World First."[3] It took another three years before the first birth of a baby that had begun life as a frozen embryo.

The Center for Surrogate Parenting in Beverly Hills does a big business in frozen embryos. They are shipped to them from around the world, transported in a special container "shaped something like a bullet,"[4] and implanted in "surrogate" mothers in California.

Freezing embryos has become a routine part of the IVF process. Like any new tool or technique, freezing was introduced as a way to improve technological efficiency and effectiveness and increase production. In this case, the product is babies. The medical rationale for freezing embryos is that the drugs given to superovulate women — to produce all those eggs in the first place — interfere with the process of implantation. If the embryos are transferred back during a non-medicated cycle, there may be a greater possibility of success. In fact, the high failure rate of IVF has not substantially changed. What has changed are the sources of human life, with "stockpiles" of "surplus" frozen embryos now "banked" in freezers around the world.

"Fertility" drugs were also introduced into IVF to improve the dismal success rate. A woman's ovaries normally release one mature egg per cycle. This complex process is coordinated by the production and secretion of a series of hormones that also prepare the womb to receive the fertilized egg. In IVF, the regulation of these hormones has been taken over by drugs and doctors. Their pharmacological fine-tuning results in more ripe follicles being ready on schedule — the clinic's schedule. As Australian Doctor Alan Trounson, one of many doctors who began his career with animals and moved to women, puts it, "If you're going to follow the woman's own natural ovulatory schedule and let her do the whole thing alone, you need to have operating tables available at your beck and call. You need to have staff that are on call all the time to obtain the eggs.... So if you can take over all that by just giving the girls [sic] an injection, you've really achieved something in terms of the cost of the procedure."[5]

There are other costs though, costs that Dr. Trounson has not factored in. The use of fertility drugs poses both known and suspected health risks to the women who take them and to any children they may produce. They are not insignificant and may include higher rates of ovarian cancer,[6] and the risk of developing a condition known as ovarian hyperstimulation that, in its most extreme form, can be fatal. Women have died from IVF. This fact is seldom reported in the "medical miracle" stories. Babies are not exempt from this reproductive experimentation either. IVF and the use of fertility drugs has sent the multiple birth rate soaring.[7] The more babies, the greater the chance of prematurity — as high as 94 percent in triplet, quadruplet or quintuplet pregnancies[8] — and the greater the health problems that fall on those babies (See Laura Sky in Volume Two).

The cost of abandoning these drugs would be too great for those with a vested interest in the reproduction business. Ares-Serono, a multi-national drug company known more commonly as Serono, is a major manufacturer of "fertility" drugs. Serono has been described as "the only company aggressively addressing the needs of millions of people with fertility problems."[9] Meeting those "needs" netted Serono $260 million in 1991.[10] But Serono doesn't just sell drugs. In 1989 it acquired Bourn Hall, the IVF clinic set up by Patrick Steptoe and Robert Edwards, the two men known as the "fathers" of the first IVF baby. Today, Bourn Hall is considered the largest IVF clinic, research and teaching centre in the world. Through their "not-for-profit educational" arm, Serono Symposia, Serono runs training courses and conferences for doctors, nurses, pharmacists and patients, and puts out "educational" pamphlets, brochures and video tapes. Perhaps most insidiously, it has well developed links with organizations of the infertile in Canada and the U.S. Given the relationship of these groups to Serono it is not surprising, but nonetheless distressing, that their public positions resemble promotions for the infertility industry more than anything else.[11]

While IVF doctors remain unsuccessful in producing live, healthy babies, they have managed to make thousands of "surplus" embryos. Now, whoever produces the embryo controls the way it is used. For the first time, scientists have virtually unlimited access to human embryos for research and experimentation. Some of this research has been directed toward producing an array of new tools and techniques in an effort to "improve" IVF and expand its markets. Micromanipulation and zona drilling (making an opening in the wall of the egg) make it possible for technicians to insert sperm directly into the egg. Male-factor infertility is now considered a "medical" indication to use IVF on women. A number of IVF clinics around the world, including one in Canada, offer pre-implantation diagnosis of the embryo. The "precision genetics and personalized service" that United Breeders boasts of in their colourful brochures has now become part of the business of human reproduction.

In the U.S., IVF is a growth industry. A recent *New York Times* article (in the *Money* section), documented a steady increase in IVF clinics from less than 50 in 1986 to 180 in 1990.[12] I visited one of those clinics in Pasadena, California. At the Huntington Reproductive Center, Dr. Paulo Serafini sells pre-implantation sex selection of the IVF embryo to couples who want to "complete" their family with a baby of a specific gender. When I asked him where he learned this new technique he smiled and said, "Neal First."

I'd heard that name before. In 1989, I had gone to Israel, to the 6th World Congress on In Vitro Fertilization and Alternative Assisted Reproduction. On day three, there was a session on genetic analysis of the pre-embryo and even though it started at 8:30 in the morning, the hall was packed. It was the hot topic of the conference. With this technique, reproductive medicine was no longer limited to the treatment of infertility. The ability to biopsy and evaluate cells from a human embryo had made genetic experimentation a part of human procreation.

One of the speakers at that session began his presentation with a slide showing three identical-looking cows. He was Neal First. He works at the University of Wisconsin, in the Department of Meat and Animal Science. He clones cows. Every spring he also runs a training session in his barns for members of the American Fertility Society, for doctors like Paulo Serafini.

"Test tube" babies, "frozen" embryos... no one seems to think twice anymore about these technological transformations of life. But people want to know about cloning. The idea of making multiple copies of the same creature seems to fascinate and repel us in equal measure.

Last winter, I was part of a panel on the reproductive technologies and the future. A man in the audience asked a question about cloning. The IVF doctor on the panel was very dismissive of the question. He said that cloning had nothing to do with human reproduction, and those who said it did were guilty of irresponsible scare mongering!

I had a different answer. I told the man who asked the question about Neal First and the IVF conference in Israel. With nuclear transfer — the proper name for the kind of cloning he does — First had developed techniques for manipulating and diagnosing embryonic material, tools that doctors like Serafini were already using for pre-implantation diagnosis of human embryos.

Dr. First describes nuclear transfer as "a powerful tool for studying embryo development [and] providing identical research animals [which would] allow production, selection and sale of high performance cloned cattle, sheep and perhaps swine."[13] Cloning cattle is already commercially applied to increase access to, and the availability of, a "desirable" product. Those same techniques make it possible to offer — or in the U.S., sell — pre-implantation diagnosis: a service that may provide couples with the possibility of having a baby of the desired gender or genes.

And the IVF doctor on that panel was wrong about cloning and human reproduction. I guess it is hard to keep up, even if you are in the trade. Only eight months later, in October 1993, front page headlines announced the successful cloning of human embryos in the United States using exactly the same techniques the cattle docs use to produce those identical cows.[14]

New technologies cost a lot of money to develop and implement. No one could afford to pursue them without the possibility of reward down the road. Cloning as a means of producing domestic animals is already paying off. And the same techniques that produce multiple copies of cows or sheep are also being used to make transgenic animals — super species, genetic elites used to improve breeding programs. "Pharming" uses genetically engineered animals as living production plants, drug factories that provide scientists with pharmaceutical proteins produced in their milk. And in a new field called "xenografts," pig embryos are injected with human genes so their hearts, livers and kidneys can be used as transplants for humans. The future is a rich one.

Carrying out pre-implantation diagnosis on human embryos also costs money. The start-up costs of the EPICS (Early Pre-implantation Cell Screening) program at the University Hospital in London, Ontario were covered by a grant from a private foundation. It didn't cost the government any money but it also removed the possibility of open discussion in the political arena about whether or not this technology should be pursued or invested in. Jeffrey Nisker thinks it should. He runs the EPICS program. He sees this as cost-effective technology. His screening program would reduce the number of children born with disabilities, saving the state money it would have spent on their care. This cost-benefit analysis of human worth comes with the technological package.

People with a new product are always looking to expand their potential market. It makes good business sense. In the spring of 1993, at a conference on prenatal diagnosis in Toronto, Dr. Nisker implied that pre-implantation diagnosis could become a standard part of the IVF procedure. Then every IVF baby could be, as Abby Lippman wryly noted, "GOOD" (Genetically Ordered and Optimized Descendant).[15]

In September 1990, the first international symposium on pre-implantation genetics was held in Chicago. Cow-man Neal First was at this conference too, but mice were the favoured research animals this time. Advances in the techniques of embryo micromanipulation, DNA amplification and gene transfer in lab animals have enormous implications for human reproduction. These tools don't stay in the mouse labs for long as was evident at the Chicago conference. Not content with simply diagnosing the embryo, scientists are gearing up for the next technological step, human germ-line genetic manipulation — adding foreign genes to the developing human embryo and producing genetic changes that would be passed along to subsequent generations.

These days, lawyers follow technological developments as closely as they follow ambulances. At the Chicago conference, The American Bar Association (ABA) presented its "ethics" position on germ-line gene "therapy." "Experimentation with, or treatment by, human germ-line gene intervention which results in changes of the genetic information should be done only in an institution licensed by an appropriate federal agency."[16] The ABA position represented a common perspective at this gathering, one that had already gone beyond asking "should we do this," to "how do we do it?"

More than once while doing research for my films, I spoke with scientists who didn't seem to know that their work had already moved from mice to people, from cows to women.

Janet Rossant makes transgenic mice at the Samuel Lunenfeld Research Institute of The Mount Sinai Hospital in Toronto. She uses genetically altered mice to make models of human diseases. I went to see her after the pre-implantation diagnosis conference in Chicago.

Rossant was surprised to hear that there was enough work going on in human pre-implantation diagnosis to warrant a conference. I showed her the *Journal of In Vitro Fertilization and Embryo Transfer* where the abstracts from the conference had been published. There was an even mix of scientists working with mice and with women. Some of them worked both sides, transferring what they had learned from mouse to human embryos and back. Rossant was particularly alarmed by the American Bar Association's statement. As far as she is concerned, there is no good scientific reason for ever doing germ-line "therapy" in humans no matter how seemingly careful the ethical rational is. It is not a position shared by most of the scientists at that conference. Their work is fuelled by the pursuit of the possible and the profitable and the only limitations are the technical ones.

The speed with which new tools are being developed and technical limitations overcome astonishes even those inside the field.

In a recent issue of an international biotech magazine, the "product of the month" was a Molecule Transfer System. There are several models available. The system is used to make transgenic animals. It makes them better — "a transfer efficiency of 200 embryos per minute for the system, compared with two embryos per minute for microinjection" — and faster, "total time required to process 1000 eggs, is 5 minutes, compared with 500 minutes required using microinjection."[17] And while it doesn't say so in the article, it probably also makes them cheaper.

Feminist concerns about pre-implantion diagnosis as a stepping stone to germ-line manipulation are often dismissed by those who tell us that the technical problems are insurmountable. They obviously aren't reading the right trade journals. But then, most scientists seem to read very little beyond a narrow slice of their own field. It is a variation of the "I just make these little widgets, I don't make bombs" approach to the world. We've seen where that has gotten us in the past.

One of those reproductive widgets is a technique called *in vitro* maturation of oocytes. When it is bovine oocytes they are after, the ovaries of cows are removed at the slaughterhouse, the eggs sucked out and brought to maturity in the lab, and then used to make embryos. "The technique has proved its worth as a means of obtaining much cheaper embryos from abattoir ovaries for all aspects of our experimental program. The systems provide controlled access to the stages of oocyte maturation and embryo development that are vital to understand if current cloning techniques are to be improved and if bovine stem cell production is to be mastered en route to controlled transgenesis in livestock."[18]

I met Keith Betteridge, the man who wrote that text, at his research centre at The University of Guelph, Ontario Veterinary College, Department of Biomedical Sciences. Betteridge experiments on cows. He showed me the opening in the wall where ovaries freshly collected at the abattoir are passed into the lab. I asked him how he felt about the same technique being used in human reproduction, with women's eggs. He turned to me with an expression I call the "Oh, no. Not another off-the-wall feminist" look! "There is no application in human reproduction," he told me rather brusquely. So I pulled out of my briefcase a file I carried everywhere I went. It is my *in vitro* maturation file, and none of the items in it have to do with cows. I showed him a newspaper article from a British paper. The headline read, "Fertility Treatment Could Use Ovaries From Dead Women." In the article, Robert Winston, director of the

Reproductive Unit, Hammersmith Hospital, London (where, by the way, the first clinical program in pre-implantation diagnosis was implemented) is quoted as saying that *in vitro* maturation was "exciting and important and could be a solution to the problem of egg donation. The idea of using ovarian tissue which has been discarded for other reasons would be a tremendous advance and be extremely useful." The expression on Betteridge's face changed.

I could have shown him the clipping from another British paper headlined, "Babes From After Death Moms" or one from a Montreal paper, "Fetuses Would 'Mother' Children." That one described using *in vitro* maturation techniques on ovaries removed from female fetuses, gaining access to their nearly one million "primitive" eggs. A team in Scotland is gearing up to transfer ovaries from fetuses into infertile women and those "past childbearing age" — always looking for new market opportunities! (See Lippman in Volume Two.) As the doctor in charge of the project modestly notes, "It would be a precedent to have a dead fetus as the genetic mother of a child."

Betteridge would have recognized that technology. Using fetal eggs is another technique being developed in the bovine world, and already being transferred to women, and human reproduction. To really comprehend the impact of the reproductive technologies we have to understand them as an interrelated cluster of techniques. Yet of all the tools being sharpened by the reproductive scientists out there, I think *in vitro* maturation is the most dangerous. This technique will give scientists access to unlimited numbers of eggs and open the way to the production of human embryos on an industrial scale. Potential human beings will be produced in the same way as lab mice and cattle are and, eventually, for the same reasons, "to produce more and cheaper embryos or progeny of desired genotypes."[19]

One day, when we stop and ask ourselves how this happened, how human procreation became another industrial process, we will follow the technological trail back to IVF. We will see how *in vitro* maturation was marketed as an "IVF breakthrough," a "development that could vastly reduce the costs, complexity and discomfort...and lead to a vast simplification of *in vitro* fertilization."[20]

Efficiency, speed and cost-effectiveness. These are the values of technology and now they are the values of human reproduction. And this is how *in vitro* maturation and the new cloning technique are being sold: just more tools to improve IVF, to guarantee that it can really deliver.

Technology transfer doesn't flow just one way. Women were the mammalian research subjects used for the development of *in vitro* fertilization, a technique that is only now finding commercial applications in the cattle industry. Most bovine embryos are still created *in vitro* and retrieved through embryo flushing.

Experimentation with superovulation in cows began in the 1930-40s. But even now, "one of the most persistent weak links in the ET (embryo transfer) chain is the unpredictability of donor's response to superovulation."[21] Taking advantage of the experimentation that has been conducted on women, animal reproductive scientists are using some of the same techniques to improve the effectiveness of superovulation in their four-legged patients. These include taking chemical control over the cows' own hormonal system and, as in IVF programs, "an injection of human chorionic gonadotrophin (hCG) to induce ovulation in a controlled fashion."[22] After years of "profiting" from technologies researched on cattle, we can now give something back to the cows by treating them like women!

Serono is one of the major manufacturers of hCG. They market it under the brand name of Profasi. In a booklet they provide to their customers about "fertility" drugs they suggest that women, "Try to relax and do nonstressful, fun things during their drug treatments." Maybe if the farmers could figure out what a "fun thing" is for a cow, they could improve their success rates.

There are some benefits in these shared reproductive experiments. The literature produced by the animal biotech scientists provides us with an evaluation of technological risks that is hard to obtain when women are the research subjects.

In the *Journal of Reproduction and Fertility,* a paper on the superior value of embryos produced from fetal eggs (bovine in this case), notes that "the [fetal] ooyctes would never be exposed to the environmental influences that they encounter in the adult ovary... These might include exogenous hormones used to promote growth, lactation or superovulation, physical factors such as irradiation resulting from nuclear accidents, ultrasound used for diagnostic purposes, or known toxins that have been identified in human follicular fluid. Avoidance of these influences could be beneficial to animal breeding programs."[23] And presumably, our own as well!

* * * * *

I like the country; I like animals and some day, I'd like to raise sheep. Maybe that's why I found the visits to the barns where they experimented on animals so difficult. I spent one day at a bovine research center in Quebec. We drove out to a dairy farm nearby. There were frozen embryos in the back of the truck. I was talking with the young woman sitting next to me about embryo flushing. She is a veterinary technician and she performs that particular procedure on cows all the time. She didn't know that "uterine lavage," as medical doctors like to call it, was also being done to women. It was quite a surprise to her. She knows it hurts the cows. She does it to them.

I've never read anything about what uterine lavage feels like included in any of the literature on the subject. It hasn't come up when I've heard doctors talk at conferences, either. The technique is pretty much the same though. In one presentation a doctor showed slides — first of cows, then of women. They were both posterior shots, and the tubing looked pretty much the same. All the women in the room squirmed.

Embryo flushing has been used for years in bovine reproduction for both commercial and experimental purposes. Top quality cows are superovulated, artificially inseminated with the sperm of prize bulls and the resulting embryos are washed out of their bodies. The embryos are transferred into recipient cows of lesser commercial value, who are often chemically synchronized to receive the embryos. It is really not surprising that the first guys who thought they could flush embryos from women and make money from it were two American cow men. Dick and Randy Seed (you couldn't get away with inventing names like that), own a successful cattle breeding business. In the early 1980s the Seeds brought together an IVF doctor, John Buster, and an investment banker, Lawrence Sucsy, and went into business. Women were recruited with the sales pitch that they would be helping infertile couples to have a child. These initial "donors" were paid about $100 per embryo flushing.

The first baby to have begun life in the womb of one woman and to be gestated in another was born at the Harbor-UCLA Medical Center in California in January, 1984. John Buster was the doctor, Lawrence Sucsy raised the money, and the experiment was financed by the Seed's company, Fertility and Genetics Research Inc.

Gena Corea, in her book *The Mother Machine,* documents the risks women face from embryo flushing. If the fertilized egg is not washed out, the "donor" could be left pregnant or suffer an ectopic pregnancy that could destroy her own fertility. She is susceptible to pelvic infection from the lavage. She could also contract a venereal disease or even AIDS after artificial insemination with sperm from the recipient's husband.

Gena Corea quotes a member of the International Embryo Transfer Society as saying, "I don't think the cow has ectopic pregnancies... That's one of the worrisome aspects of trying to take a technology developed in one species and apply it to another."[24]

Uterine lavage never quite paid off as the Seed brothers and their investors had banked on. But embryo flushing is experiencing a second wave of interest as a new market opportunity opens up. And not surprisingly, it has nothing to do with infertility and everything to do with genetics.

Currently, pre-implantation diagnosis is done on one, maybe two cells removed from a four- to eight-cell human embryo. But as the techniques of DNA amplification and evaluation expand, scientists want more cells to work with than they are able to get from those embryos created *in vitro.* Later stage embryos, called blastocysts, have lots and lots of cells, but they will not grow for long in petri dishes. They have to be taken from women's bodies. They have to be flushed out.

John Buster and Lawrence Sucsy both attended The First International Symposium on Pre-implantation Genetics in Chicago in 1990. John Buster was in Chicago as part of a team from the University of Tennessee. The work they presented at that conference rates as perhaps the most cynical manipulation of women as experimental subjects that I have ever encountered. Their published abstract is a model of doublespeak. Entitled, "Recovery Of Blastocysts By Uterine Lavage Following Superovulatory Drugs," it begins, "Uterine lavage allows noninvasive recovery of human blastocysts. Blastocysts are uniquely suited for microbiopsy and pre-implantation genetic diagnosis." It goes on to complain that they have been having a tough time getting enough blastocysts from women they have been flushing in spontaneous cycles. So following the lead taken in cattle where, "the yield of bovine embryos obtained by uterine lavage increases greatly when superovulation is performed," they "administered ovulation induction agents to women wishing to donate embryos to infertile couples."

Now this experiment had nothing to do with infertility. No embryos or blastocysts were ever transferred to infertile women. Sandra Carson, one of the Tennessee group, told me that herself. Yet 15 women aged 21 to 40 who had answered ads claiming to offer help for the infertile, were subjected to one of four experimental superovulation regimes, and lavaged one to three times daily for five to ten days! Helping the infertile was simply a pretence for this reckless treatment of women. And I have no doubt it isn't over, because the abstract concludes, "alterations in ovulation induction, insemination timing or lavage technique are under continued investigation to increase blastocyst yield and hopefully fulfil the potential of uterine lavage for pre-implantation diagnosis."

Those women in Tennessee were guinea pigs in an experiment that could determine how all women may be expected to reproduce some day. I have heard Robert Edwards chide a room full of doctors for not working hard enough to develop uterine lavage so that the flushed, evaluated — and eventually genetically improved — embryo could become the norm in human reproduction. Hand-in-hoof, commerce and medicine, industry and science are taking us step by step in that direction.

Elizabeth Olsen knows a lot about superovulation, embryo transfer and sex selection. She farms with her son and husband in Bow River, Alberta. In September, 1990, as president of The Women of Unifarm, the provincial farm women's organization, she wrote and presented a brief to The Royal Commission on New Reproductive Technologies.

The women of Unifarm have a very particular perspective on this technological encroachment into human procreation. They use reproductive technologies as part of their every day lives. It isn't easy being a farmer in Canada and those techniques can help them maximize their herds, maybe keep them from going under. But she knows that women are not cows.

In her brief, Elizabeth Olsen wrote, "Recognizing that we as lay people do not have the background in medicine (science), theology, law or philosophy, our organization however has some very real concerns about the directions in which the new reproductive technologies are taking us. We are going to work at these issues as seen through our experiences as agricultural producers in the changing world of plant and animal production. There are parallels which can be drawn.

"We certainly measure the value of stock on the farm, by their ability to reproduce healthy young. If that is not the case, the animal is sold. Surely we cannot and should not view human reproduction in the same way. There are certainly farmers who look after the 'runts' among their animals even though they recognize the non-profitability of such an action. Can we as a human society, do any less in caring for those who are disabled in any way?"[25]

* * * * *

I went to the country to write this piece. I can look out the window and see cows grazing in the field that belongs to the small dairy farm down the road. That farmer's family has been there since the turn of the century. He is an old man now and the farm will go when he does. I think of him as Old MacDonald.

Maybe we want a world where super-cows only leave their stalls to be flushed or "pharmed?" Maybe we want a world where only genetically enhanced babies get made by scientists for the people who can afford them? But I don't see anyone asking us. In the meantime, scientists and doctors, lawyers and ethicists, businessmen and investment bankers are forging ahead making the kind of world that suits their interests. If it doesn't suit ours, we had better act now.

NOTES

1 *On The Eighth Day: Perfecting Mother Nature.* Film one, *Making Babies,* film two, *Making Perfect Babies.* Distributed in Canada by the National Film Board.

2   Deborah Tennant, "Fighting the crisis of infertility," the *Globe and Mail*, Monday June 21, 1993.

3   Gena Corea, *The Mother Machine. Reproductive Technologies from Artificial Insemination to Artificial Wombs*. New York, Harper and Row, 1985.

4   Interview with Bill Handel, The Center For Surrogate Parenting, Beverly Hills, California. From the film, *On The Eighth Day: Perfecting Mother Nature*. Part one, *Making Babies*.

5   Corea, Gena. *The Mother Machine*.

6   Gutfeld, Rose, "FDA Says Label Of Fertility Drugs Must Warn Users," the *Wall Street Journal*. January 14, 1993; The U.S. Food and Drug Administration announced that the drug companies that make Pergonal and Clomid had to add to their labels a warning about the possible link between these drugs and ovarian cancer.

7   Rod Mickleburgh, "Rising rate of multiple births creates burden for taxpayers," the *Globe and Mail*, Wednesday January 6, 1993. The rate of multiple births among women using *in vitro* fertilization is 23 times that of women conceiving normally.

8   *Ibid*

9   Alison Leigh Cowan, "A Swiss Firm Makes Babies Its Bet." the *New York Times*, April, 19, 1992.

10   *Ibid*

11   Deborah Tennant, the *Globe and Mail*.

12   Alison Leigh Cowan, "A Swiss Firm Makes Babies Its Bet," the *New York Times*, April 19, 1992.

13   Neal First, "Nuclear transfer." Abstract from 6th World Congress on In Vitro Fertilization and Alternative Assisted Reproduction.

14   Gina Kolata, "Scientist Clones Human Embryos, and Creates an Ethical Challenge," the *New York Times*, October 24, 1993.

15   Abby Lippman, Letter to the *Canadian Medical Association Journal* commenting on their February 15, 1993 article on the EPICS program.

16   Sherman Elias, and George Annas, "A Place for Germ-Line Therapy?," *Journal Of In Vitro Fertilization and Embryo Transfer*. Volume 7, Number 4, August 1990.

17   *Biotech Products International*. Volume 5, no. 3/4. April 1993.

18   K.J. Betteridge, "Embryo Research at the University of Guelph: An Update."

19   K.J. Betteridge, "Embryo Transfer in a Biotechnical Age," October 1990.

20   Richard Saltus, "Korean doctors report in-vitro fertilization breakthrough," the *Boston Globe*, Wednesday November 15, 1989.

21   K.J. Betteridge, "Embryo Research at the University of Guelph: An Update."

22   *Ibid*

23   K.J. Betteridge, C. Smith, R.B. Stubbings, K.P. Xu and W.A. King, "Potential genetic improvement of cattle by fertilization of fetal oocytes in vitro." *Journals of Reproduction and Fertility*. Suppl. 38. 1989.

24   Gena Corea, *The Mother Machine*.

25   Elizabeth Olsen, Submission to The Royal Commission on New Reproductive Technologies by the Women Of Unifarm. September 14, 1990.

8

FROM REPRODUCTION TO MAL[E] PRODUCTION: WOMEN AND SEX SELECTION TECHNOLOGY

Sunera Thobani

What has the white, male lawgiver to say to any of us? To those of us who love life too much to willingly bring more children into a world saturated with death? Abortion, for many women, is more than an experience of suffering beyond anything most men will ever know; it is an act of mercy, and an act of self-defense.

Alice Walker[1]

The words of Alice Walker acquire more poignancy when considered in light of the sex selection technology which uses abortion for purposes of "selecting" male fetuses. What can be more painful than the abortion of a fetus solely because it is the same sex as the woman who carries it? What can teach a woman more profoundly to internalize the devaluation of all women in patriarchal society?

In a period which has been described as a "backlash" against women by even liberal standards (Faludi, 1992), the extent of the attacks on the limited gains made by the women's movement has been fierce. Sexual violence, as well as other forms of violence against women, are increasing globally. This violence is linked to the right wing attack on women's demands for economic, social and political equality. The use of sex selection technology for the purposes of not "selecting" female children, therefore, can only be understood as part of this attack on women in the wake of the gains made by the women's movement over the past few decades. And, as the reproductive process becomes a profit making enterprise, it is the women most marginalized by the relations of race, class and gender who become the major focus of the attack.

This paper examines how the opening of a sex selection clinic which targeted the South Asian community in British Columbia, Canada, merged the dynamics of capital, science and technology into a relationship which refashioned racist, class and patriarchal power relations. This merger was realized in the commercialization of a new reproductive technology for misogynist use which thereby strengthened the ongoing oppression of women.

SEX SELECTION TECHNOLOGY

Sex selection technology is one of the new reproductive technologies. It allows for the selection of the sex of a fetus prior to birth. In general, there are two approaches to sex selection: pre-conceptional and post-conceptional. The pre-conceptional techniques allow for selection to take place prior to fertilization of the egg. Laboratory processes are employed in an attempt to separate sperm carrying an X chromosome from those carrying a Y chromosome and a woman is subsequently artificially inseminated with the "right" sperm to produce a fetus of the "desired" sex. These approaches, despite their technical refinements, are not all that "selective," raising the probability of the "desired" sex only to about 70 percent from the 50 percent it would have been without any intervention.

These odds are considerably greater with what has been, until recently, the most commonly used approach to sex selection: post-conceptional. This approach relies on screening techniques such as amniocentesis, ultrasound and chorionic villus sampling (CVS) to determine the sex of the fetus. If the fetus is found not to be of the "desired" sex, it is aborted.[2]

In the medical literature, sex selection is said to have three different purposes: (1) for "medical" needs, i.e., to prevent the transmission of sex-linked genetic conditions; (2) for "family completion," i.e., to provide a child of a different sex than a couple's previous offspring; and (3) for "pure" sex selection.[3] What is interesting in this categorization is that none of the purposes are (strictly) medical. Even the decision to prevent the birth of human beings with certain genetic-linked conditions is not purely a "medical" one, but a moral and political one. Likewise, the term "family completion" is generally applied only to "western" families who, it is claimed, do not necessarily prefer one sex over the other, but desire only a "balanced" family. Instead, it is only in relation to peoples of colour that the purpose is presented as what it really is, sex selection, pure and simple. In consequence of this categorization, the "crude" sex selection practised by peoples of colour is set apart from the more "sophisticated" family completion ideals and "medical needs" of the "western" family.

Yet, whatever the purpose, sex selection must be understood as part of a eugenic dynamic in a society that facilitates selective breeding. Studies indicate that in the overwhelming majority of cases, it is female fetuses who are aborted after a pregnant woman undergoes post-conceptional sex selection. These observations reflect the marked "preference" for male offspring that has been documented in multiple surveys and reports from a number of countries, all of which show the preference for male children cuts across racial and cultural divisions. Wherever they have been studied, preferences "almost universally favour boys."[4]

For practical purposes, therefore, sex selection works to facilitate male selection. And this should come as no surprise given the power relations in capitalist society. That men are valued more than women is a fundamental tenet of patriarchal societies, notwithstanding the fact that certain classes and races of men are valued above other classes and races (Davis, 1983). Statistics which indicate that women own 1 percent of the property in the world, that women earn an average of 60 cents to every dollar earned by a man, that women are the poorest of the poor, and that horrifying numbers of women are subjected to abuse and violence, only make this preference for males clearly visible at all levels of society. Sex selection reflects, as well as perpetuates, the devaluation of women.

`OPPORTUNITIES UNLIMITED... YOUR TIME IS LIMITED, SO PLEASE DON'T WAIT...`[5]

In the summer of 1990, an Australian doctor named Stephens based in California (where he already operated three clinics and a toll free line) announced the opening of a sex selection clinic, Koala Labs., in Blaine, Washington.[6] Koala Labs. was a commercial venture and, like the sex selection clinic operating in Scarborough (Ontario) since September 1987, which charged $600 for the initial insemination and $500 for subsequent inseminations,[7] it planned to charge $500 (US) for the test.

Blaine is about 40 km from Vancouver, and Vancouver has a sizeable South Asian population. Calling on South Asians in British Columbia to take advantage of "opportunities unlimited," the Koala Labs. clinic intended primarily to serve this community. The initial advertisement for the clinic appeared on August 17, 1990 in a publication serving the South Asian community called *The Link*. It prompted a number of letters from women's organizations demanding its withdrawal[8]. *The Link* responded by pulling the advertisement, admitting it to be in bad taste. Claiming he could detect the sex of a fetus as early as 12 weeks into pregnancy, Dr. Stephens then launched a sophisticated marketing campaign in *India Abroad, Tasvir*, as well as the previously mentioned paper, *The Link*. The advertisements appeared in both Punjabi and English, as did mailings to gynecologists in the area, and direct mailings to 10,000 households. Flyers were also distributed around the Main and 49th Street area known as "Punjabi Market," which comprises mainly South Asian businesses and stores.

What is particularly interesting is the manner in which Dr. Stephens initially presented his reasons for opening the clinic, as well as his subsequent defense of it. Claiming his technique was a "godsend" for South Asian women in a letter to The Royal Commission on New Reproductive Technologies, the doctor explained that "East Indian" women are "terrified" of having more females because "East Indian families want to be assured of having male babies."[9] Arguing that South Asian culture condones this preference for males, he went on to say:

What I have found with [people of East Indian origin] is that they use me to diagnose sex. If it is discovered that it is a female, it is always the girl that they want to select to undergo foeticide.... Why should I cut my own financial throat? Why should I have to go out on my own to change their cultural attitudes?[10]

The doctor claimed he had been approached by a number of South Asian male doctors to open the clinic, and that some of the men had already brought their wives to him. There exists an "underground network" of South Asians who have used his services in North America, he informed a reporter.[11] The clientele at the clinic in Blaine was defined in the following terms:

Nearly all are immigrants from India who have settled near Vancouver. Nearly all are under cultural pressure to produce male heirs. And nearly all will have abortions if they learn the babies they are carrying are girls.[12]

Discussion about the clinic subsequently focused squarely on South Asian "culture" and the doctor's representation of the South Asian community played a significant role in shaping the public discourse as it was expressed and reported extensively in the media. Moreover, the implicit notion, often made explicit by the doctor, that South Asian culture celebrates and condones this particular form of misogyny remained unchallenged in the media, which focused primarily on understanding these "cultural" attitudes. Thus, a number of letters and opinion pieces published in newspapers railed against immigrants who bring their "cultural" practices to Canada, as did a number of callers to radio programs. In one of the more bizarre pieces, a writer cited figures of selective abortions at a clinic in Bombay, going on to relate these figures to the South Asian immigrant community by claiming, "This is the cultural attitude many immigrants bring with them here." Arguing that Dr. Stephens is something of a visionary, the author goes on to praise the doctor:

Far from condemning Dr. Stephens, we should give him a medal for offering something that may help save the world from overpopulation, raise the status of women and, not incidentally, give parents a choice in the gender of their offspring.[13]

It is a curious logic which leads this particular writer to argue that the selective abortion of female fetuses would raise the value of females in society, as well as help curb overpopulation in the Third World.[14] That the doctor himself cited no such laudable goals, although he repeatedly defended his financial interests, makes this piece all the more intriguing.

Even respectable news programs such as CBC's *The Journal* were not immune to the "cultural backwardness" argument. The report on sex selection aired in November, 1990, and repeated in January, 1991, focussed mainly on the clash between "ancient" cultural values and "modern" science. The report included film from a party given by a South Asian family to celebrate the birth of a son. And although the report mentioned that some families also gave parties to celebrate the birth of a daughter, the program chose to show only the party celebrating the male child.

Although studies consistently indicate that the preference for males exists in many communities, the public discussion aroused by the Koala clinic focussed only on the South Asian community. The 1990s are a period when mounting racist violence has been documented in the United States, Canada and Europe indicating a rising level of racial hostility against immigrant communities. In such a climate, the sole focus on the South Asian community by the doctor who opened the clinic, as well as the subsequent public discourse as shaped by the media, ensured the vulnerability of this community to increased racist hostility.

This identification of sex selection with the South Asian community also served to obscure how the practice of sex selection poses a threat to the future of women in all communities. Although in this particular instance the new clinic targeted the South Asian community, the use of sex selection technology crosses racial and cultural divides. Sex selection technology is used to further the devaluation of women, which has become a global phenomenon. Hence this technology ultimately has an impact on the lives of all women.

It also serves to hinder any analysis of women's oppression as resulting from power relations in society and shifts the focus away from the economic, social, political and legal structures which shape this inequality. The framing of the public discourse resulted in the South Asian community and its culture becoming the focal point of attention, and the very pertinent questions of the use of modern science and technology for misogynist and racist purposes were sidelined.

The stereotyping of South Asian culture as the only one which condones male selection also worked to single out South Asian women as passive victims, thereby weakening the analysis of the common experiences of all women in Canadian society as defined by their inequality. Feminists have argued that the devaluation of women globally is best addressed by analysis of how power relations are structured within a system stratified along gender, race and class hierarchies (hooks, 1984; Davis, 1983; Mies, 1986). Women are devalued in every community in Canadian society today, as the statistics on the rape, abuse and poverty of women show. By isolating the South Asian community as inherently oppressive toward women, the colonial definition of the "backwardness" of peoples of colour was invoked, as was the necessity to adopt mainstream "Canadian" (read western) values to end this oppression. Furthermore, this particular definition of "cultural" difference was grounded in racial difference, i.e., mainstream "Canadian" culture versus immigrant, South Asian culture, with the latter assumed to have timelessness, unchangeability and inherent backwardness, characteristics previously affixed to notions of racial difference.

This particular doctor drew upon a persisting racist definition of South Asian culture that first took root in western civilization at the time of the colonization of India. The "backwardness" of "traditional" societies in the Third World was a justification colonizers used to defend the continued domination of "their" colonies. Arguing the superiority of western values and the European race, the colonizers took upon themselves the necessity of "modernizing" colonized peoples even as they were exploiting them to further the interests of colonizing societies. The racism which exists in Canadian society maintains this sense of superiority and by invoking the stereotype of the "cultural" practices of South Asians, and by defining this in a monolithic and uniformly misogynist manner, the South Asian community became the target not only of the doctor's campaign, but also of racist hostility in the larger society.

On the other hand, the provision of this very "modern" scientific technology enabled patriarchal relations within the South Asian community to be perpetuated and strengthened. Whether the South Asian men the doctor claims approached him actually did so cannot be verified. However, that some members of the community have availed themselves of this service, and defend its provision, is beyond question. CBC's *The Journal* report included an interview with a South Asian woman who chose to remain anonymous while defending the services offered at Koala Labs. In a world where the oppression of women is defended as a necessary, and sometimes even desirable, state of affairs, any number of pressures can be brought upon women by family and community members to undergo sex selection and to bear sons. The error would be in defining this selection as "choice." Surely such "choices" call more for an analysis of how women are made to internalize the devaluation of women, particularly the devaluation of women of colour.

The relationship between capital, science and technology, in the form of commercialized sex selection ventures, gives the patriarchal devaluation of women scientific and medical legitimacy, as well as prescribes a misogynist set of practices in the name of "culture." In this particular instance, racist forces from outside the South Asian community, and patriarchal forces from within the community, were both strengthened as a result.

INSTITUTIONAL RESPONSES TO SEX SELECTION

At the time the Royal Commission on New Reproductive Technologies held hearings in Vancouver, Koala Labs asked for an appearance in defense of the clinic. Fifteen women's organizations supported a demonstration, organized by the India Mahila Association, to protest the clinic. The demonstration was held outside the hotel while the hearings were underway. A number of immigrant women's groups, including South Asian women's groups, also presented a brief to the Commission in which they called for a ban on sex selection technology and urged the Canadian government to work with others to enforce an international ban. The National Action Committee on the Status of Women (NAC), representing over 500 women's organizations across Canada, also called for a ban on sex selection.

Pointing out that preferences for males exist cross-culturally, the brief presented on behalf of the Immigrant and Visible Minority Women (B.C.) stated:

> If women are devalued in our culture, then we also have a strong tradition of resistance to this devaluation of women. Culture is a dynamic social process, not static and mechanistic as racist stereotypes try to imply even as they impose reactionary, oppressive practices upon us. We are opposed to having technologies directed against our communities that devalue women further and which are being legitimized in the name of culture and tradition. We are opposed to this stereotyping of the Indo-Canadian culture and here today represent that tradition of resistance which is firmly rooted in our culture and which has fought against the devaluation of women for centuries.[15]

Whatever hopes the women's organizations had that their concerns would be taken seriously were quashed upon reading the Commission's subsequent report, which stated, "Some presenters said that women may also be pressured into aborting female fetuses because of a cultural preference for male offspring...."[16] The report called for "culturally appropriate" services for immigrant communities.

The Commission was also quick to draw a line distinguishing between "Canadian" couples who would use sex selection for "family completion" and "ethno-cultural" communities who would use the technology simply for sex selection. "Canadian" couples would use the technology to "equalize" their families, and not in any discriminatory manner, the Chairperson concluded.

Although the Commission has yet to produce its final report and recommendations, the public statements made by the Commission thus far do not bode well for women. By choosing to focus on "cultural sensitivity," and working with a patriarchal, racist interpretation of South Asian culture, the mutual re-enforcement of racist and patriarchal relations will be at the expense of South Asian immigrant women. While the Commission calls for "culturally appropriate" services to meet the needs of immigrant communities, it has not engaged in a discussion of the particular interpretation of South Asian "culture" towards which it is calling for "appropriateness" and "sensitivity." Indeed, by referring to sex selection only in terms of "cultural" preferences, the Commission is paying little heed to the voices of South Asian women, and is exhibiting its willingness to work with the rigidly patriarchal prescription of culture.

The Society of Obstetricians and Gynaecologists of Canada (SOGC) has also issued a policy statement on sex selection. The recommendation it makes echoes the comments made by the Chairperson of the Royal Commission, stating support for sex pre-selection in the case of the transmission of genetic disorders, as well as under research conditions for family completion purposes.

The results of these recommendations set a double standard for the use of this technology: when "Canadian" (i.e., caucasian) couples use the technology, it will be considered non-discriminatory and will be referred to as "family completion"; and when South Asians use this technology, it will be considered an inevitable consequence of their misogynist culture and will be referred to as "sex selection." Thus are the lines being drawn between the acceptable use of the technology by "modern," "civilized" mainstream society, and the deplorable use of it by "backward," "misogynist" immigrants.

THE PRO-CHOICE MOVEMENT AND REPRODUCTIVE RIGHTS

While a number of South Asian women's organizations were active in opposing the clinic from the time of the initial announcement of its opening, a significant moment in the controversy was the entry of the pro-choice movement in British Columbia into the discourse on sex selection. In a provocative piece in *The Province*, a journalist defined sex selection as raising "a prickly dilemma for pro-choice advocates."[17] The pro-choice advocate this particular journalist interviewed defended a woman's right to choose in the following words: "She must always have the freedom to terminate a pregnancy for whatever reason, no matter how abhorrent that may be to others."[18]

While the pro-choice advocate refrained from speaking on behalf of South Asian women, and also did not speak to the issue of South Asian culture, the larger question remained unaddressed. Having fought for abortion rights on the basis of abortion being a woman's "right to choose," the pro-choice movement was being confronted with women supposedly "choosing" to abort female fetuses. Could "choice" therefore be defended even when that choice furthered the devaluation of women?

This question has implications extending beyond the preference for males, for sex selection is not the only form of selective abortion currently being practised. The aborting of fetuses who have been defined as having disabilities poses a similar dilemma. Can feminists defend selective abortion on the basis of a woman's right to "choose," when these "choices" reflect the dominant society's devaluation of certain groups of people, i.e., women, people with disabilities, people of colour, etc.?

With the developments in pre-conceptional sex selection, the larger question becomes even more complex. The impetus for the provision of pre-conceptional sex selection sometimes arises from anti-abortion sources. Anti-abortion groups might be opposed to selective abortion, but might very well support pre-conceptional sex selection on the basis that it furthers "choice" and avoids abortion. In fact, a South Asian doctor who subsequently announced his interest in opening a sex selection clinic in Vancouver in August, 1992, did so on this very basis. "The abortions really disturbed me," this doctor said. "I felt that there should be an alternative technique. I feel a woman should have choice."[19]

The rhetoric of "choice" can therefore be used against women in furthering provision of technologies which actually encourage women to "choose" to participate in their own devaluation.

Initially reluctant to address the issue other than expressing support for South Asian women, the B.C. Coalition of Abortion Clinics (B.C.C.A.C.) remained silent on questions of "choice" and "culture." However, a number of South Asian women have been active within the abortion rights movement in

British Columbia, and in their dialogue with both the pro-choice activists and labour organizations at a number of rallies and public events,[20] these women have argued that the discussion of sex selection has to shift from the terrain of "cultural" attitudes and "choice" into the arena of how the inequality of women is structured in society.

The question of "choice" has been addressed by women of colour active in the struggle for abortion rights for at least two decades. Critiquing the "pro-choice" position as reflecting the narrow white, middle-class experience of women who have access to resources which enable them to make "choices," women of colour argued that they have struggled for abortion rights not on the basis of "choice" but on the basis of equality rights and the need to gain control over their bodies and their lives.[21]

These ongoing dialogues, both historical and contemporary, resulted in a moment of alliance between South Asian feminists and feminists from other communities. Along with the publicity generated over the Royal Commission and the recognition in the women's movement that new reproductive technologies increased the patriarchal control over women's bodies, the dialogue begun over sex selection led to a conference held in the summer of 1992, sponsored by the B.C.C.A.C. The conference identified the need for a national anti-racist feminist movement which would address the question of abortion rights within the context of reproductive rights and acknowledged the necessity for feminists of colour to play a leadership role in this movement.[22]

Whether that acknowledgment will translate itself into action in the mainstream women's movement remains to be seen, but South Asian women's organizations in British Columbia successfully organized against the opening of a sex selection clinic in Vancouver in 1992,[23] as well as organized resistance to the clinic in Blaine.

CONCLUSIONS

The opening of the sex selection clinic in Blaine reveals how the relations of race, class and gender are constantly re-fashioned and are being perpetuated by science and technology through the commercialization of reproductive technologies. The Royal Commission's work, which will be the basis for future legislation, indicates thus far that this State-appointed body is willing to apply rigid, patriarchal definitions of "culture" to racial minority communities and to uphold the power relations of race, class and gender. Public discussions of "cultural sensitivity," without the necessary discussions of power relations in society, and without analysis of structures of domination, only serve to re-inscribe patriarchal relations. Who defines "culture," what are the vested interests in particular definitions, and what are the powers which enforce particular interpretations on communities is contested terrain. In the case described here, the definition of South Asian culture was imposed upon the community by external forces acting in tandem with the patriarchal forces within the community. This definition of culture worked against the interests of South Asian women, creating more barriers in their struggles for equality.

By choosing a racist and patriarchal definition of South Asian culture, both racist and patriarchal structures are strengthened in the name of "cultural sensitivity," thereby furthering the oppression of South Asian women. Indeed, to the extent that sex selection technology is used cross culturally, it serves to further the devaluation of all women.

At a moment when South Asian women are questioning and challenging patriarchal interpretations of culture and tradition, acceptance of a misogynist definition of culture becomes even more problematic. The result, in this instance, is the use of very "modern" technologies and "advanced" science in the service of "ancient" structures of domination and oppression. A report prepared for Canada's Royal Commission on New Reproductive Technologies warns that:

> ...there will no doubt be changes in the new reproductive technology which will likely make sex selection cheaper, earlier, and perhaps more accurate. Such advances are likely to make sex selection even more common than it already is. And there is a huge potential demand for such technologies.[24]

Despite the attempts to scapegoat the South Asian community in British Columbia, sex selection technology continues to pose an increasing threat to the rights of all women.

BIBLIOGRAPHY

Ahmed, L. *Women And Gender In Islam*, Yale University Press 1992.

Burstyn, V. "Making Perfect Babies," *Canadian Forum* April 1992.

Canadian Research Institute for the Advancement of Women [CRIAW], *Our Bodies... Our Babies?*, 1989

Conseil du Statut de la Femme, *Dilemmas*, Quebec Undated.

Corea, Gena. *The Mother Machine*, Harper & Row, New York 1979.

Davis, Angela. "Goodbye to the Universal Woman," transcribed by Roxana Lee, *Kinesis*, Vancouver March 1990.

Easton, Shelly. "Dr. Accused of Racism, Sexism," the *Province*, Vancouver November 27, 1990.

Faludi, Susan. *Backlash: The Undeclared War Against American Women*, Crown Publishers, Inc., New York 1991.

Griffin, Kevin. "Campaign Promotes Female Fetus Abortion, Critics Say," the *Vancouver Sun*, Vancouver September 19, 1990.

Goodman, E. "Sex selection by abortion repugnant," the *Vancouver Sun*, Vancouver January 5, 1990.

Harding, S. (ed.) *Feminism & Methodology*, Indiana University Press 1987.

Hartmann, B. *Reproductive Rights And Wrongs*, Harper & Row, New York 1987.

hooks, b. *From Margin to Center*, South End Press 1984.

Hossie, L. "Gender by Choice, and guess which one?" the *Globe And Mail*, Canada August 14, 1992.

Matheson, Graeme. "What's wrong with choosing your baby's sex?" the *Globe and Mail*, Canada December 3, 1990.

McCune, Shane. "Pre-natal sex ID poses dilemma for choicers," the *Province*, Vancouver November 28, 1990.

Merchant, Carolyn. *The Death of Nature*, Harper & Row 1983.

Mickleburgh, R. "Doctor to defend fetus sex test in B.C.," the *Globe and Mail*, Canada November 15, 1990.

Mies, Maria. *Patriarchy and Accumulation on a World Scale*, Zed Books, London 1986.

Muha, Laura. "A Doctor's Prenatal 'Pandora's Box'," *San Francisco Chronicle* December 16, 1990.

O'Neil, R. "Reproduction committee strife gives birth to skepticism," the *Vancouver Sun*, Vancouver November 18, 1991.

O'Neil, P. "'Embarrassing' infighting brings call for probe," the *Vancouver Sun*, Vancouver December 10, 1991.

O'Neil, P. "Feminists' bias cited in firings," the *Vancouver Sun*, Vancouver December 17, 1991.

Patel, Vibhuti. "Sex-Determination and Sex-Preselection Tests in India: Modern Techniques for femicide," *Bulletin of Concerned Asian Scholars*, Vol. 21, No. 1, Boulder 1989.

Royal Commission on New Reproductive Technologies, "What We Heard: Issues and Questions Raised During The Public Hearings Ottawa September, 1991.

SOGC, Policy Statement, No. 15 November, 1992.

Stackhouse, J. "An Indian couple's dilemma: 'Girls are very expensive'," the *Globe and Mail*, Canada August 14, 1992.

The Link, Letters to the Editor, Vancouver September 21, 1991.

The *Vancouver Sun*, Editorial, Vancouver September 20, 1990.

The *Voice*, Editorial, Vancouver #3, 1990.

Thobani, S. "From Reproduction to Mal(e)Production: The Promise of Sex Selection," *Ankur*, Vancouver April/May/June 1991.

Thobani, S. "Position Paper Presented on Behalf of the Immigrant & Visible Minority Women (B.C.) to the Canadian Royal Commission on New Reproductive Technologies," Vancouver November 1990.

Thobani. S. "Making the Links: South Asian Women and the Struggle for Reproductive Rights," *Canadian Woman Studies*, Vol. 13, No.1 Fall, 1992.

Todd, Douglas. "Checking of Fetal sex Defended," the *Vancouver Sun*, Vancouver (Nov. 27, 1990).

Vines, Gail. "Old wives' tales `as good as sperm sorting'," *New Scientist* January 30, 1993.

Wigod, R. "Birth Research Extended," the *Vancouver Sun*, Vancouver July 9, 1991.

Wigod, R. & O"Neil, P. "Panel member says no split despite lawsuit," the *Vancouver Sun*, Vancouver December 7, 1991.

NOTES

1   From *Nation*, 22 May, 1989. Quoted by Rosalind Pollack Petchesky in *Abortion And Woman's Choice*, Preface, Northeastern University Press 1990.

2   For an excellent listing of some of the new reproductive technologies and their descriptions, see the Kit put together by The Canadian Research Institute for the Advancement of Women (CRIAW), *Our Bodies... Our Babies?* 1989.

3   These three purposes are clearly outlined in the Policy Statement prepared by the Canadian Fertility and Andrology Society and the Society of Obstetricians and Gynaecologists of Canada. The Policy Statement was issued in November, 1992.

4   L. Hossie, "Gender by choice, and guess which one?" the *Globe and Mail*, Canada August 14, 1992.

5   Quoted from an advertisement for Koala Labs. which appeared in the newspaper, *The Link*, Vancouver August, 1990.

6   Subsequently, it was reported that this doctor had previously applied to Grace Hospital in British Columbia to practice the technique he had patented in the U.S., but had been turned down. The technique, is called FASA ("Visualizing of the fetal external genitalia in early pregnancy by fetal anatomical sex assignment").

7   The CRIAW Kit on New Reproductive Technologies, *Our Bodies... Our Babies?*, 1989 mentions the opening of this clinic by a Dr. Allan Abramovitch.

8   "MediaWatch" and the "Immigrant and Visible Minority Women of B.C." were among these women's organizations.

9   R. Mickleburgh, "Doctor to Defend fetus sex test in B.C.," the *Globe and Mail*, Canada November 15, 1990.

10 Kevin Griffin quotes doctor Stephens in "Campaign promotes female fetus abortion, critics say," the *Vancouver Sun*, Vancouver September 19, 1990.

11 Dr. Stephens was reported to have said this by Kevin Griffin in "Campaign promotes female fetus abortion, critics say," the *Vancouver Sun*, Vancouver September 19, 1990.

12 Quoted from the *San Francisco Chronicle*, December 16, 1990.

13 The author of this piece is Graeme Matheson, the title of the piece is "What's wrong with choosing your baby's sex?," published in the *Globe and Mail*, December 3, 1990. Mr. Matheson is described as "a writer and editor living in Vancouver."

14 An examination of the racism which underlies arguments about Third World overpopulation and the necessity of controlling the procreation of Third World peoples is beyond the scope of this paper, and suffice it to note other authors have addressed this.

15 S. Thobani, Position Paper Presented On Behalf of The Immigrant and Visible Minority Women of British Columbia to the Canadian Royal Commission on New Reproductive Technologies, Vancouver November 1990.

16 The Royal Commission on New Reproductive Technologies, What We Heard: Issues and Questions Raised During the Public Hearings, September 1991.

17 Quoted from Shane McCune's piece in the *Province*, "Pre-Natal sex ID poses dilemma for choicers," Vancouver November 28, 1990.

18 McCune quotes a member of BCCAC in his piece in the *Province*, "Pre-natal sex ID poses dilemma for choicers," Vancouver November 28, 1990.

19 Cited from a report in the *Vancouver Sun*, "Sex-choice doctor under peer scrutiny," Vancouver September 5, 1992.

20 This dialogue took place, among other venues, at a rally organized by B.C.A.C.C. in October, 1991, and an evening public event jointly sponsored by B.C.C.A.C. and the B.C. Federation of Labour in Spring, 1992.

21 For further discussion, see an interview with Angela Davis, "Goodbye to the Universal Woman," transcribed by Roxana Lee, *Kinesis*, Vancouver March 1990 and Thobani, S. "Making the Links: South Asian Women and the struggle for Reproductive Rights," in *Canadian Woman Studies*, Vol. 13, No. 1 Fall, 1992.

22 This alliance has to be understood within the ongoing work that feminists of colour have been doing within the mainstream, white women's movement, in Canada for decades. That such alliances are actually being forged in some areas stands as testimony to the effectiveness of the questioning of the mainstream women's movement by women of colour in their commitment towards an anti-racist feminism.

23 In August 1992, a South Asian doctor based in Toronto announced his interest in opening a sex selection clinic in Vancouver. The resulting protest by feminists generated enough publicity to involve the College of Physicians and Surgeons, whose inquiry into the ethics of such a clinic have proved to be a deterrent to the opening of the clinic thus far.

24 L. Hossie, "Gender by choice, and guess which one?" the *Globe and Mail*, Canada August 14, 1992.

9

THE NEW REPRODUCTIVE TECHNOLOGIES, PUBLIC POLICY AND THE EQUALITY RIGHTS OF WOMEN AND MEN WITH DISABILITIES

Sandra A. Goundry

For The Canadian Disability Rights Council

Women and men with disabilities have an enormous stake in the way in which public policy is formulated with respect to the promotion and application of the new reproductive technologies. The Canadian Disability Rights Council (CDRC) has examined the claims made about the new reproductive technologies — to reduce the incidence of disability and expand the range of reproductive choices for women — and pronounced them misleading, suspect and dangerous.[1]

The first claim is misleading given that the vast majority of disabilities have causes which are not genetically related; it is dangerous because of the negative implications of eugenic thinking for existing persons with disabilities. The second claim is suspect given the introduction of the new reproductive technologies into a social context in which disability-based discrimination and sex discrimination are pervasive; it is dangerous because, in the present context, the new reproductive technologies actually restrict the range of choices available to women with disabilities specifically and non-disabled women generally. Thus, insofar as the new reproductive technologies serve to entrench disability-phobic attitudes and promote eugenic thinking, they devalue the lives of persons with disabilities and undermine their equality aspirations.

At the same time, it is clear that women with disabilities are doubly affected by the new reproductive technologies as both sexism and disability-based discrimination profoundly affect their lives. As reproductive autonomy is a cornerstone of women's equality aspirations, all women, including women with disabilities, need to insure that the new reproductive technologies will not erode that autonomy but will, instead, enhance their reproductive choices.

CDRC's research has demonstrated that the implications of the new reproductive technologies for persons with disabilities are almost wholly negative — given their introduction into a disability-phobic and sexist society. Indeed women and men with disabilities and non-disabled women are among the groups who stand to be most fundamentally affected by the technologies. It is to these individuals and groups that we must look for guidance as to how to formulate public policy which is respectful of the equality aspirations and human rights of women and men with disabilities and non-disabled women. CDRC has developed a number of guidelines and a set of principles to assist in the formulation of public policy with respect to the new reproductive technologies.

RESPECTING THE DIGNITY AND EQUALITY ASPIRATIONS OF PERSONS WITH DISABILITIES

IDENTIFY AND REMOVE THE EUGENIC COMPONENT

In the context of medical interventions in human reproduction, eugenic thinking is pervasive; that is, the focus is on the production of "perfect babies." It is alarming that little or no thought is given to the consequences of embarking on the slippery slope of this technological "Brave New World." Somewhere lost in the discussion is the question of whether a society of genetically "cleansed" individuals is a worthwhile societal objective — not to mention questions concerning the use of eugenic-based thinking to get there. The passive acceptance of the new reproductive technologies is extremely alarming to persons with disabilities who have already experienced many different forms of oppression and brutality in the name of eugenics.

Eugenic practices historically have been used in attempts to rid society of "socially undesirable elements." What characteristics are labeled "socially undesirable" change over time and place. In Nazi Germany, Jews, persons with disabilities and gays and lesbians were given this label and, as a consequence, were systematically sterilized and exterminated. Women and men with disabilities, particularly mental disabilities, have been similarly labeled in recent times in North American society and have been sterilized, institutionalized and otherwise isolated from mainstream society as a result. This predilection for eugenic thinking is dangerous given the ease with which the designation of "undesirable" is attached and the consequences which result. Members of all disadvantaged groups are particularly vulnerable to these kinds of discriminatory attitudes.

Current practices associated with prenatal screening and diagnostic technologies underscore the extent to which eugenic values are operating in their promotion and application. Eugenics is operating every time a woman with a disability is discouraged from considering motherhood, every time pressure is put on a woman with a disability to undergo screening during her pregnancy, every time a woman, whether disabled or not, is expected to abort a fetus with a disabling condition, with the list of "detectable disabling conditions" ever growing.

The very fact that extensive use is being made of diagnostic testing during pregnancy to detect, for the purpose of elimination, a variety of disabling conditions is evidence that a eugenic bias is operative. The presumption that a positive test result will inevitably be followed by an abortion is particularly repugnant to and disrespectful of people with disabilities. This eugenic presumption is being acted upon as indicated by the fact that approximately 90 percent of "positive" amniocentesis tests result in the termination of "wanted" pregnancies. These figures are sending out a warning signal.

The message about disability is loud and clear — the prospect of having a disabled child is simply not acceptable or feasible for many prospective parents. The message to all women is equally clear: it is not socially acceptable to carry to term a fetus which has a disabling condition.

The agenda of the detection technologies is unabashedly eugenic. With the emphasis on the production of "perfect" babies, the implicit message of the new reproductive technologies is that disabilities can and should be weeded out of the population by eliminating fetuses which exhibit certain "defective" traits. This twentieth century version of eugenics, which casts disability as an inherently bad thing, is being introduced into an already disability-phobic society wherein disability-based discrimination is pervasive. In this context, giving birth to anything other than a "perfect" baby becomes not only "undesirable," but preventable, and therefore irresponsible.

Thus far CDRC's research suggests that the emphasis on eliminating disability through the new reproductive technologies, without addressing the social context in which they are being promoted and applied, has a number of disastrous implications for persons with disabilities; namely this perspective:

1. disregards the fact that most disabilities are not genetic in origin;

2. directs resources away from eliminating environmental causes of disability and from providing supports for existing persons with disabilities;

3. diverts attention from the role of societal structures in the oppression of persons with disabilities;

4. ignores the extent to which disability is a social construct;

5. entrenches disability-phobic attitudes and leaves discriminatory practices intact.

Despite the negative ramifications of this form of contemporary eugenics for existing persons with disabilities, little attention has been devoted to naming the eugenics bias of the new reproductive technologies for what it is and taking steps to remove it. Predictably, the perspective of persons with disabilities has not been accorded much weight in public policy discussions. The task then, for public policy-makers, is to identify the eugenics bias and determine if, and how, these technologies can be applied in a disability-positive manner. Only then can the new reproductive technologies be introduced in a way which is respectful of the dignity and equality rights of persons with disabilities.

REDISTRIBUTE RESOURCES TO ADDRESS NON-GENETIC CAUSES OF DISABILITY AND PROVIDE ADEQUATE SUPPORT SERVICES FOR EXISTING PERSONS WITH DISABILITIES

One of the claims made on behalf of the new reproductive technologies is that the incidence of disability in the population will be reduced. This claim is made despite the fact that most disabilities are *not* genetic in origin and with complete disregard for the approximately 3 million existing Canadians with disabilities. The truth is that the principal causes of infant disability are poverty-related (ie. inadequate nutrition of pregnant women) and many disabilities are acquired later in life because of workplace and vehicular accidents, violence, environmental hazards and the natural process of aging.

Yet rather than address those causes of disability related to poverty or exposure to toxic environments or unsafe workplaces, hundreds of millions of dollars are being poured into technologies which target only a very small portion of disabilities. (It is noteworthy that this wrong-headed approach is not limited to the "detection" technologies. The focus of the so-called fertility-enhancing technologies is also misplaced as millions of dollars are channelled into fertility clinics without addressing the fact that the causes of infertility are largely environmental or medically induced.)

In this context, claims to reduce the incidence of disability are also made without regard for the general well-being of the millions of Canadians with disabilities. State resources which are being funnelled into the new reproductive technologies could be utilized to dismantle disability-based discrimination and raise the standard of living of Canadians with disabilities through providing funds to deliver adequate support services. Those support services would include reproductive health information centres for women with disabilities.

What the public policy-makers have to remember is that the new reproductive technologies represent a billion dollar industry which has an enormous financial stake in diverting our collective attention from the non-genetic causes of disability AND from providing adequate support services for existing persons with disabilities. The agenda of the reproductive technology industry must be rejected outright as a blueprint for the formulation of public policy and the determination of resource allocation by the Canadian government.

TACKLE DISABILITY-PHOBIC ATTITUDES OF THE NON-DISABLED MAJORITY

The new reproductive technologies are informed by the scientific and medical communities' perspective of "disability as defect." This discriminatory perspective serves to foster and perpetuate the prevailing societal view of people with disabilities as persons to be pitied as enduring tragic lives which are not worth living. As long as discriminatory language is used to refer to people with disabilities (as well as fetal anomalies), disability-phobic attitudes will be reinforced. The use of disability-positive language is a pre-requisite to dismantling these disability-phobic attitudes and perceptions.

This pejorative view of disability, subscribed to by the non-disabled majority, is based on its inexperience with and ignorance of disability and what it means to live with one. It is a view which ignores and invalidates the experience of people with disabilities. Persons with disabilities have repeatedly informed the non-disabled majority that it is not the disability per se which restricts their attempts to participate fully in society. Rather it is the social stigma attached to disability and the legal, physical, economic and social barriers to participation which prevent persons with disabilities from leading full, productive lives. In this sense, disability is largely a social construct.

If the voices and experiences of persons with disabilities were given more weight, more attention and resources would be applied to removing the social, legal and economic barriers to participation. As a result, more persons with disabilities would be able to lead full and productive lives which help to dismantle stereotypes and misconceptions.

THE GATEKEEPERS TO THE NEW REPRODUCTIVE TECHNOLOGIES NEED TO HAVE A BALANCED PERSPECTIVE ON DISABILITY AND SHOULD BE REQUIRED TO PRESENT THAT INFORMATION IN A DISABILITY-POSITIVE MANNER

The relationship of women and men with disabilities to the medical establishment has been marked by a litany of abuses including forced sterilization, dangerous drug "therapies," electro-shock and institutionalization. This history is relatively recent such that the new reproductive technologies, in the hands of a medical establishment which still views disability as "defect," are unlikely to be used in a way which would ameliorate their condition of disadvantage.

Like everyone else, members of the medical community are products of a disability-phobic society. They are also engaged in a profession which has a hostile view of disability. The bias against disability is reflected in the medical terms for fetal anomaly which include "defective," "deformed" and "abnormal." Despite their negative view of disability, it is members of the medical community who have control over the application of new reproductive technologies. Members of the medical profession decide which "conditions" warrant detection and elimination. Further, general practitioners and genetic counselors are charged with the dissemination of information about the new reproductive technologies and decide when, on whom, and how they should be used.

This situation requires fast and immediate attention. The educational curricula of medical and other professional schools must be informed by balanced information. Continuing education programs must be developed which tackle disability-phobic attitudes and provide practitioners with accurate, up-to-date, balanced information on disability. Then the onus must be placed on these professionals to deliver this information to patients and clients, non-disabled and disabled, in a way which is respectful of the equality aspirations of people with disabilities and mindful that the purpose of the information is to enhance women's decision-making around reproductive issues.

EQUAL ACCESS TO REPRODUCTIVE HEALTH FOR WOMEN (AND MEN) WITH DISABILITIES

Women and men with disabilities want equal access to reproductive health information. Discriminatory attitudes held by the non-disabled majority dictate that women and men with disabilities are not considered appropriate parents. The same attitudes and ignorance are responsible for the fact that women with disabilities are denied access to information about sex and birth control and are consistently discouraged from giving birth or parenting. For these reasons the demand for equal access to reproductive health counseling for women and men with disabilities is warranted.

There are at least two discriminatory biases operating in relation to the access issue. The first is that women with disabilities which are genetic in origin should be denied the opportunity for reproduction as a matter of public policy because they are "high risk" in terms of producing a child with a disability. The implicit message is "we don't want more people like you." The second is the biased assumption that people with disabilities do not make good parents — a stereotype which attaches particularly to persons with mental disabilities. Women with mental disabilities are hardest hit as they are unlikely to fit this society's conception of the "ideal woman/mother." The key is that these biases are *discriminatory* and to the extent they are used to bar access to reproductive health services, they are contrary to the existing human rights law and therefore illegal.

All criteria that restrict access to reproductive health counseling have to be reviewed for discriminatory biases — criteria based on disability, family status, income levels, ethnic background and sexual orientation are automatically suspect as discriminatory. Further, such criteria are likely to have a disproportionate effect on women with disabilities as more than one of these criteria may apply.

ENHANCING THE REPRODUCTIVE AUTONOMY OF ALL WOMEN

ADOPT A FEMINIST PERSPECTIVE WHICH RECOGNIZES THAT REPRODUCTIVE AUTONOMY HAS A PARTICULAR MEANING FOR WOMEN WITH DISABILITIES

Clearly, women with disabilities stand to be doubly affected by the new reproductive technologies as both sexism and disability-based discrimination profoundly affect their lives. In this light, to ignore the feminist perspective on new reproductive technologies is to discount the lives of that 51 percent of the disability rights movement which is made up of women. For the most part, women with disabilities share the concerns of non-disabled women with respect to the implications of new reproductive technologies and insist that a feminist perspective be adopted by public policy-makers.

The new reproductive technologies represent an unprecedented surge in the medicalization of women's reproductive lives. Women's control over their bodies is attenuated as medical personnel decide that ultrasound should be applied routinely in hospitals, amniocentesis should be "strongly recommended" for women 35 years of age and over for the purpose of detecting Down syndrome and surgical interventions in the birthing process are in everyone's best interest. Similarly, genetic screening for fetal anomalies is presented as a medical and social imperative.

This trend of increased medical intervention in women's lives continues despite the fact that the long-terms risks of these technologies have not been studied. The bottom line remains that women with disabilities must take control and able-bodied women need to retain control over decision-making in regard to these technologies.

It is important to understand though, that for women with disabilities, "reproductive rights" and "new reproductive technologies" have a particular meaning — a meaning which has been informed by a historical experience of oppressive attitudes and discriminatory practices in relation to their sexual and reproductive lives. Forced sterilization and the prescription of unsafe contraceptives have marked the lives of generations of women with disabilities. In short, the exercise of reproductive autonomy has not been part of the historical experience of women with disabilities which is a product of the fact that they are both women and disabled.

For women with disabilities, the new reproductive technologies do not enhance their reproductive autonomy mainly because these technologies are introduced into a disability-phobic society where sexism is pervasive. Thus, for women with disabilities, reproductive rights mean more than access to birth control and the right to abortion. It also includes:

* freedom from nonconsensual sterilization;
* the right to accurate, balanced information about reproductive health and disability;
* the right to refuse prenatal testing;
* the right to carry to term a fetus identified as having a disability;
* the right to adequate social and financial support for raising a child with a disability; and
* the right to equal access to fertility-enhancing technologies.

These rights if given effect will serve to enhance the reproductive autonomy of all women.

INFUSE THE LANGUAGE OF CHOICE WITH REAL MEANING BY INCLUDING THE CHOICE TO HAVE A BABY WITH A DISABILITY

Reproductive autonomy is enhanced when women are empowered to make informed decisions about their sexual and reproductive lives absent any kind of coercion. The language of choice has particular resonance for women as it symbolizes the long-standing struggle for abortion rights. But the language of "choice" has been misappropriated by the proponents of the new reproductive technologies. It is not clear at all that the new reproductive technologies have expanded the range of choices for all women. Rather CDRC's research suggests that in the context of the new reproductive technologies, "choice" has little meaning for women generally and women with disabilities in particular. Rather it is used to disguise eugenic practices and construct "empty" choices. The eugenic component of the new reproductive technologies has been outlined earlier.

The "choice" is empty because it is often made in an immediate context which is coercive and a societal context which is disability-phobic. The immediate context is the genetic counseling session; the societal context encompasses all stages of women's lives. With respect to the immediate context, the coercive element must be removed. For example, women have reported enduring very negative videos on Down syndrome as part of their "counseling." This is coercive. What women require is accurate and balanced information about disability and the opportunity to at least talk about raising a child with a disability with those who have had direct experience doing it. Otherwise, all of the available options are not clear.

Of course, one genetic counseling session which provides accurate, balanced, disability-positive information to a woman is unlikely to strip away attitudes developed after absorbing years of disability-phobic messages. This is why the CDRC is adamant that disability-based discrimination and bias must be tackled at all levels of society so that the option to have a baby with a disability is a real one. Further, "balanced information" in and of itself will not provide access to the financial resources and support services necessary to raising a child with a disability. These resources must be made available. For both women with disabilities and non-disabled women, "choice" has no meaning unless the right to "choose" includes the real, practical option of having a baby with a disability.

ENDORSE AND INCORPORATE THE CONCEPT OF INFORMED CHOICE INTO THE PROMOTION AND APPLICATION OF ALL NEW REPRODUCTIVE TECHNOLOGIES

The only way to enhance the reproductive autonomy of women with disabilities is to recognize that they have the same information needs as non-disabled women in relation to their sexual and reproductive lives. Like non-disabled women, women with disabilities want and need accurate, balanced information, tailored to their particular circumstances, about safe and reliable contraception, safe sex, birthing, abortion, prenatal screening and the fertility-enhancing technologies — so that they are in the position to make their own decisions with respect to reproductive health.

The concept of informed choice must apply to all decisions both women with disabilities and non-disabled women make concerning their reproductive health. For women with disabilities, this is extremely important to recognize as their struggle for reproductive autonomy is premised on gaining recognition of the fact that they are sexual and reproductive beings. Women with disabilities want this recognition and the responsibility for determining their own reproductive health needs.

In relation to counseling, informed choice means that all women receive effective, unbiased, non-directive counseling for all aspects of their reproductive and sexual health. For genetic counseling to be effective, women require accurate, comprehensive information, about the rate of occurrence of diseases, the risks involved in testing, the predictive value of the tests a woman is considering, the range of options open to her and the costs and available resources involved — presented in a comprehensive, understandable fashion. To be unbiased, the educative component of counseling has to be emphasised, with a view to empowering women to make real choices based on all the information at their disposal and which do not necessarily conform to prevailing societal attitudes about children with disabilities. Accurate, balanced information about disability which goes beyond a medical perception of disability must be made available to all women, including women with disabilities.

CONCLUSION

Women and men with disabilities have an enormous stake in the way public policy is formulated with respect to the promotion and application of the new reproductive technologies. CDRC's research has demonstrated that the implications of these technologies, taken as a whole, for persons with disabilities are almost wholly negative. This conclusion comes from a recognition that the new reproductive technologies are being introduced into a society which is both disability-phobic and sexist.

Given these concerns, CDRC recommends that a set of principles be developed to inform public policy in relation to the new reproductive technologies — principles which reflect respect for disability equality rights and sex equality rights as guaranteed by the Canadian Charter of Rights and Freedoms. This set of principles must provide the philosophical basis for removing the eugenic component from the new reproductive technologies and for enhancing women's reproductive autonomy. The principles include:

1. The true measure of the value of the new reproductive technologies lies in the extent to which they can benefit the individuals and groups who are most directly affected by them, that is, women and men with disabilities and non-disabled women.

2. The promotion and application of the new reproductive technologies can only be undertaken in a way which supports and enhances the dignity, respect and equality aspirations of women and men with disabilities.

3. A feminist perspective should be adopted to focus policy analysis on ensuring that the reproductive autonomy of both disabled and non-disabled women is enhanced by the new reproductive technologies. It is important to recognize that for women with disabilities, reproductive autonomy has a particular meaning.

4. Reproductive health counseling must be made available on an equal basis to all who want access as human rights principles apply to the delivery of these services.

5. Disability rights and sex equality rights are not opposed where all women, especially women with disabilities, are given full control over their own bodies and reproductive autonomy and where they are given the opportunity to make choices based on accurate and disability-positive information. At the same time it must be recognized that disability rights and sex equality rights are both advanced if discrimination against persons with disabilities is eradicated.

6. A fetal rights approach should be resisted as detrimental to both disability equality and sex equality rights.

NOTES

This piece is largely a summary of the Canadian Disability Rights Council's (CDRC) Final Brief to the Royal Commission on New Reproductive Technologies (July, 1992) which was prepared by the same author in consultation with an advisory group. All of the 22 Recommendations have been removed as well as specific references to the Royal Commission. The CDRC is a national, non-profit, organization designed by people with disabilities to advance the equality rights of disabled Canadians. The CDRC promotes the rights of people with disabilities through legal education, legal research, and test case litigation. New reproductive technologies and their impact on the equality rights of people with disabilities is a major concern and priority issue to the CDRC. The CDRC's head office is located at #208 — 428 Portage Avenue, Winnipeg, Manitoba R3C OE4 and can be contacted by phone at (204) 943-4787; by fax (204)943-1223; and on DISC: CDRC.

1   See: Four Discussion Papers on New Reproductive Technologies (September 1991) prepared for CDRC and the DisAbled Womens' Network (DAWN) by Yvonne Peters, Gwen Brodsky, Maria Barile and Sandra A. Goundry with summary of the issues by Shelagh Day. It is in these Discussion Papers, which are available from CDRC, that the reader will find more detailed discussion of and references for some of the points raised in the Brief.

10

NEW REPRODUCTIVE TECHNOLOGY: THE DICHOTOMY OF MY PERSONAL AND THE POLITICAL

Maria Barile

When I began writing about the new reproductive technologies (NRTs), I began to understand just how complex and multi-dimensional the issue is. And you can be sure that when a subject that involves women's bodies — and the information the public gets about this subject is unclear, inconsistent and contradictory — most people will not have the chance to really understand what's at stake. I resolved to help change that with my writing, if not by providing answers, then at least by asking questions.

Recently I have begun to question myself. My questions are those of a woman approaching her 40th birthday who thinks about the past and wonders with confusion about the future, a future when I will no longer be part of this planet. Mine are the questions of a woman with disabilities, who, I admit, has internalized certain social and cultural myths. As a result, what I advocate politically doesn't always mesh with my personal feelings.

I realized just what that meant one day as I sat in my doctor's waiting room. Reading a letter in a magazine, I suddenly found my political ideas crashing into the realm of the personal. The letter was from a woman expressing her joy at having a child of her own using *in vitro* fertilization. For just a moment I found myself wondering what kind of a child my genes would produce. Would I have a girl? What colour eyes and hair would she have? Would she be like me? Would she be passionate about women's issues and social justice, like I am? Then again, what if I had a boy who grew up to be a chauvinist? These thoughts surfaced aimlessly in my mind, triggered by the letter from this unknown woman. There I was, for the first time, understanding, from a personal perspective, what drives women to have a child of their own at any cost.

Wait a minute! Those were my emotions speaking. Where did my logic go? My political convictions put an end to that foreboding daydream but not to the knowledge that came after it. As a disabled woman I had completely internalized the "you will not reproduce" line. The daydream made me realize just how thoroughly. But I also saw that when women have been sold the "it's your responsibility to reproduce" message, and don't have the information about IVF and the other techniques that I have, it would be so easy to be seduced. After all, I was the woman who had written so critically about these new reproductive technologies. I went back to what I had written.

I have two concerns surrounding the techniques that seem to be replacing natural procreation. The first is that they can be used to remove women's control over their bodies. The biological functions which operated individually in every woman's body will be replaced. The right to choice that we as women have won will be reclaimed not only by the men we may choose to have in our lives, but also by the male-dominated political arena that has already pronounced itself through medical and legal mechanisms. History has shown us that our rights over reproduction can be used to further the political aims of certain elites. This ranges from passing laws that outlaw abortions and legalize sterilization to laws that oblige families to limit themselves to a set number of children.

The second concern is based on an economic argument: The technology of reproduction is a rapidly growing commodity that will favour certain economic groups over others. For instance, if one pays for a surrogate mother and artificial insemination, those with money will be in a position to dominate those without; the latter will then find themselves in a position to be exploited.

Another economic consequence of the NRTs concerns women with disabilities. Regardless of the country they are living in, these women have historically been and still are in a position of poverty and easily victimized by those wanting to test and perfect new medical procedures. We only need to look at the issues of Depo-Provera and sterilization to find examples of how we are used as guinea pigs, even before the dangers of these procedures are fully understood. In 1993, almost 10 years since the effects of Depo-Provera were called into question, the long-term consequences for women who have been injected with it remain unknown.

The message generally conveyed to the public creates the impression that the main objective of NRTs is to give people more positive and progressive options. For example, we hear that NRTs would allow people to choose the type of child they want, or allow women who could not otherwise bear children to do so. Mixed in with this message is a subtle one that impacts negatively on the human rights of people with disabilities. This subtle message implies that anyone opposing the NRTs is against a woman's right to choose.

How can non-disabled men and women who have constantly been fed misinformation about disability and persuaded to believe that the lives of persons with disabilities are "not worth living" possibly be expected to choose anything but the elimination of a fetus that would develop into a child with disabilities? This view could be assumed especially by women and men who have never had any meaningful encounters with the community of people with disabilities. How can one make choices, let alone an "informed choice," based on myth?

I believe that the choices these individuals make will be based on socially-learned negative values with respect to disability, such as the fear of socially displeasing physical features. Social dogma dictates that one must be physically able and one's body must have that athletic look. These sentiments are subtly reinforced by our economic and social system and promoted by the media. This in turn gives rise to the view that the more one deviates from society's physical and mental norms, the more undesirable one is. Therefore, according to these standards, persons with disabilities are "unwell," unable to conform to society's strict standards for physical and/or mental ability and are thus among the most undesirable.

Since the beginning of time, our social systems have been determined by our economic systems, and every economic system has promoted the view that physical desirability and productivity go hand in hand. These systems value individuals according to their ability to compete in the reproductive market place. By "reproductive" I mean both the actual physical reproduction of the next able-bodied *generation*, and the production of able-bodied replacement workers in the competitive labour market.

"Undesirables" often become dependent on the state. This gives rise to the patronizing notion that society takes care of disabled persons. Today we also hear that if you choose to have a disabled child you are responsible for all its needs. Individuals are deemed to be guilty of creating social problems, or of being socio-economic burdens. One of the main messages of the NRTs is that the problem will be eliminated through genetic manipulation, altering a person's genes to correct imperfections or introduce new traits.

The fact is that every time a society faces economic difficulties, it blames the powerless for wanting more. In the case of people with disabilities, the public has been led to believe that the cost of their support is an economic burden, that the changes we demand to have our rights cost too much money. The state claims that if they give to us, there will be nothing left for other groups. Those in power use this myth to sow conflict between groups.

That is what my political self tells me, but my sudden daydream makes me face something else. I am dealing with a wave of emotions. I feel the intense personal desire of women who want their own children. It is a real, but also socially constructed sentiment. Ever since I can remember, I have heard women, the non-disabled, tell of the rewards of motherhood. But the message that I and the other disabled women of my generation have been given is that we should not, and do not want, to have children. For "our own good," of course. I have heard pregnant women being told, "as long as the baby is healthy, it doesn't matter if it's a boy or a girl." And I ask, what does that say about me and all those like me?

These new technologies are sold to women as giving them more choice. Now they can have exactly the type of child they want. But the NRTs and their illusive choices make me fearful. The physical, the ethical and the political consequences of these technologies are uncertain. Finally it is the political I come back to. It clears away the dreams, the sentimentalism that my upcoming 40th birthday brought on. When the political realities for women with disabilities are such that those in power — the policy makers, the service providers, etc. — are no longer trespassers in our personal lives, and we can make choices that are truly our own, then our personal and political will be one and the same. Perhaps then women with disabilities can fulfil their personal dreams and have genuine reproductive rights.

NOTE

A version of this article was published in *The Canadian Woman Studies Journal/Les Cahiers de la Femme*, Volume 13, No. 4., Summer 1993.

11

BREEDING DISCONTENT (REPRINTED WITH PERMISSION FROM SATURDAY NIGHT)

Varda Burstyn

The mist clung around me as I approached the central campus of the University of Hamburg. It was a cold, dark, rainy November afternoon in 1990, two days after the anniversary of Kristallnacht, the night in 1938 when German fascists went on their murderous rampage against the Jews, a rampage whose end included the extermination of one branch of my father's family in the concentration camps. With a small group of medical students, I entered a steep lecture hall to hear an introductory speech and watch a screening of the now-notorious wartime film *Ich Klage An*, which, roughly translated, means *I Accuse*. It was made in 1941, with all the lavish production values and talent the Third Reich could command, and released as propaganda to prepare the German people for the so-called euthanasia of disabled babies, which the Nazis undertook that year as part of their program of eugenics — "racial hygiene." Throughout the Third Reich, over 5,000 babies were put to death.

In Canada, in November 1990, the Royal Commission on New Reproductive Technologies (headed by geneticist and paediatrician Patricia Baird) was in the process of conducting hearings across the country on developments in reproductive and genetic engineering. I was the co-chair of the committee of The National Action Committee on the Status of Women (NAC) responsible for making a submission to the Royal Commission, and I was in Germany to investigate the strong opposition to such engineering that had arisen there — especially from the women's movement, which was more militantly critical of these technologies than in any other place. My research had led me to the historians of fascism and to this event. As it turned out, many of the most vociferous of the German critics of reproductive and genetic engineering — feminists, natural scientists, social scientists and human-rights activists — turned out to be experts in and critics of Nazi eugenic policies. The Third Reich was a worst-case scenario against which German critics consistently weigh the benefits and losses of contemporary reproductive and genetic engineering.

The term eugenics refers to the idea that there are flaws or inadequacies in the human race, manifested in and caused by genetic abnormality; and to the practice of attempting to correct the flaws through selection and breeding. As the echoes of Kristallnacht and fog settled in my mind, the course director, medical sociologist Dr. Heidrun Kaupen-Hass introduced the guest lecturer, Udo Sierck. "Udo Sierck is a historian of Nazi eugenics," she said. "He has written four books on Nazi population policies, with great emphasis on attitudes to physical difference and physical disability. He is also a leading critic of contemporary genetic technologies."

Sierck began his lecture of introduction to *Ich Klage An* by explaining the history and policies behind the sophisticated propaganda of the Nazi film industry. He pointed out that *Ich Klage An* was seen by 16-million people in 1942, after which, in a number of cities, several hundred thousand disabled people were killed. Sierck explained that the plot concerns a woman who discovers she has multiple sclerosis, deteriorates rapidly, and finally begs her doctor-husband to help her put an end to her life. The doctor, who ultimately assists his wife in committing suicide only to stand trial, is depicted as a heroic figure. An apparently minor subplot is interwoven with the main story: the tale of a baby born with a similar though unspecified condition. The function of the film is to equate the condition of the terminally ill adult with that of the disabled newborn. The message of the subplot is simple: if euthanasia is good for the first, then it must also be for the second.

Sierck ended his lecture with a meditation on first principles. "The basic premise of eugenics is that some lives are worthy and some are not," he said. "The basic practice is the selection of worthy life on the one hand, and the elimination of unworthy life on the other. Today, eugenics — those principles of ranking and selection of life — have reappeared through the new technologies of reproductive and genetic engineering. When we decide to abort a fetus who is diagnosed with Down syndrome or spina bifida, for example, we are already making a eugenic decision."

Sierck's lecture was riveting in one completely unexpected way. Erudite and passionate, he laboured to articulate every word, which made his audience work hard, too. Because of a doctor's error shortly after his birth, Udo Sierck has cerebral palsy. His twin brother has no signs of the disease. Sierck concluded with a sobering caveat: "We have to think very hard about the essential question the Nazi experience taught us to ask. Who will draw the line between worthy and unworthy life, and on what criteria? Who will benefit? Who will lose? After all, had I been born just a few years earlier here in Hamburg, I would have been put to death with those other children. I ask you: Is my life worthy?"

A stunned silence filled the hall, then the projector rolled. As I sat in the darkness watching the images flicker on the screen I realized that my own critical positions on genetic technologies, considered "extreme" by the standards of contemporary Canadian debate, would in fact be considered "soft," naive, middle-of-the-road by many German critics. I supported tightening restrictions around the use of two prenatal diagnostic techniques considered routine these days — amniocentesis and ultrasound — and a ban on the new technology known as pre-implantation diagnosis in which two cells of an eight-celled embryo are removed for genetic testing and possible manipulation.

The confrontation by German critics of the historical experience of Nazi eugenics — from extermination camps to artificial insemination programs, from mass sterilizations and infant "euthanasia" to attempts to create embryos in a test tube — has produced a group of people who are far more hardline about the technologies than their counterparts in Canada. They are much more uncompromising about what they see as the negative trade-offs between very limited health and fertility gains from the new technologies, on the one hand, and major losses in health, fertility and human rights on the other. Sierck and others I met stressed that the trend towards what is often called the "geneticization" of disability and disease — the training of science and capital on the genetic as opposed to the social causes of disability and illness — is embodied by today's prenatal genetic technologies. But no amount of genetic screening could have prevented Sierck himself from being born with cerebral palsy, for instance. In fact, the preponderance of infant disability, some say as high as 95 percent, is not caused by genetic factors: medical accidents and error form a significant part of the causes. Low birthweight, prematurity and its attendant hazards are responsible for far more. And these relate to socioeconomic, not genetic, status. The new technologies of prenatal genetic screening — amniocentesis, chorionic villus sampling, maternal blood sampling, and now, pre-implantation diagnosis — will never be able to prevent the disabilities caused by social and medical factors. In the German critics' view, geneticization diverts attention and resources away from these causes, and paves the way for the mass acceptance, and the mass practice, of eugenics. To what extent are the Germans exceptionally clear-sighted as a result of their historical experience? To what extent are they paranoid?

In North America, we've been accustomed by and large to thinking about the new technologies as straightforward boons to humankind. In keeping with our general reverence for technology and medicine, we've welcomed their marriage in the reproductive and genetic fields on the assumption that their progeny could help us with our problems — give us babies when we're infertile, prevent or ameliorate disability and disease. Hoping that there may be relief for our pain, we have accepted the incursion of technologized medicine and the marketplace it creates into the very source points of life itself: fertile gametes, gestating wombs, genetic codes. For the most part, hard questions have been confined to specialists' circles. Whether it's ovulation-inducing drugs and Petri-dish embryos or the genetic manipulation of plants, animals, and, now on the horizon, humans, many of us have not approached these technologies as complex developments with potentially negative, as well as positive, consequences.

Though genetic sterilization of the so-called mentally disabled took place for over fifty years in various parts of North America in this century, with the collusion of mental hospitals and government authorities, we have never experienced direct, mass, state-led, militarily-enforced initiatives in the control of human reproduction. The Germans have. This more than any other factor explains why in Germany, as in no other country, mass opposition to reproductive and genetic engineering, composed of women's, ecological, church, union and scientific groups, has emerged. Over the last decade, this movement has gained followers in most of the major urban centres in Germany, and has gathered enough strength to exact, against the lobbying of the industrial sector, the passage of laws against a variety of procedures and technologies that are more restrictive than those of any other country in the world.

Many of the generation of Germans who came of age in the 1960s were haunted by the Nazi experience their parents had lived through. As they became historians, political scientists, philosophers, scientists and doctors, many undertook detailed studies of their fields during the Nazi era; when I asked Heidrun Kaupen-Hass why she started working as a medical sociologist, she said simply, "My father was a doctor at the time of the Third Reich." Though much of their work remains untranslated into English, it provides a much more sophisticated and chilling analysis of that period than the crude stereotypes, still prevalent in North America today, of sadistic Nazi scientists and brutal camp commandants. What they point out, in an insistent refrain in which the word "modernity" is uttered over and over again, is that German scientists employed by the Third Reich simply expressed and implemented beliefs and values that were held in common among scientists, industrialists and government administrators and officials throughout Europe and North America.

Dr. Ludger Wess, tall and robust, is a biologist and social scientist in his late thirties. In 1985, he left laboratory work to concentrate full time on the history of science and genetics during the Third Reich. He is the author of *The Dream of Genetics: Genetic Utopias of Social Progress*. In the library of the Medical Sociology Department at the University of Hamburg, Wess told me about his work. "What was said here in Germany about the history of science during the Third Reich, especially about biology and genetics, was that it was a misuse of science, or bad science, or not even science at all. It was important to me to know whether this was true or not. So I researched what had actually happened here in the field of genetics and especially human genetics and compared what had happened in Germany to what had happened in other countries. What I discovered was exactly the opposite of the myth," said Wess. "I found a complete collaboration between the leading geneticists and science managers — people such as Hermann Joseph Muller, Conrad

Waddington, Frederick Osborn, J.B.S. Haldane, Timofeeff Ressovsky — in the leading centres of genetic research, that is, in Germany, the United States, Great Britain and the Soviet Union."

Wess has written about the involvement of the Rockefeller and Carnegie foundations in German initiatives in genetics. Both American foundations funded projects in mass genetic monitoring, particularly for mental illness, the records of which then served as the basis for involuntary sterilization in Germany during the war years. Though of great interest, the social experiments were small potatoes compared with the potential applications of genetic understanding just over the horizon. "With Rockefeller Foundation funds," Wess said, "this international group of geneticists were hard at work on the structure of the gene. Had the war not interrupted them, they would have discovered DNA."

As he uncovered the extensive network of connections between Nazi science and mainstream genetics, Wess realized that German state scientists (by the late 1930s, these were the only ones who were working) operated from the same ideological basis as leading geneticists in other countries. "I suppose you could say that they all believed genetics should be applied to get 'better' human beings," said Wess. "They wanted to control evolution. They wanted to improve human beings. They thought human beings should be improved. They were conscious and dedicated eugenicists. All of them, not just the Germans."

By understanding how 1930s science and social Darwinist philosophies came together to create a shared eugenic view, Wess believes we can better grasp the ways in which ideology, science and technology are interacting today. He explained that during the 1930s, the fruit fly was the main object of genetic experimentation and theorization. Geneticists observed that under inbreeding conditions, and with plentiful food and an absence of predators, the flies began to produce many mutant individuals. Extrapolating directly from fruit flies to humans, geneticists were struck, not to say panicked, by what they concluded: modern conditions had allowed for the proliferation of many such degenerated mutations among humans. In 1938, certain geneticists even told the politicians in Germany that only one third of the population was fit to reproduce, and two thirds of the German population should be sterilized or prohibited from procreation. "They were really, in a way, quite mad," Wess said. "They came to believe that it was imperative to find ways to preserve healthy human stock and rid humanity of these mutations or face race catastrophe within several generations. Thus they made a new evaluation of the importance of selection. They said, 'We must proceed with a program of breeding,' and began the projects of semen banks and artificial reproduction in a test tube."

This was the "dream" of genetics — ranking humans and attempting to improve on them, as humans have done with plants and animals for millenniums. There were many ways to give nature a hand. What is known as "positive eugenics," the pro-active approach to generating "good human stock," was, according to Wess's research, favoured by the Russians. In the 1920s, Soviet geneticists tried to persuade the government to artificially inseminate 20,000 women to breed better children with the sperm of "superior" men. And there were attempts at artificial insemination in Germany during the war years as well. "But for a long time the Germans preferred 'negative eugenics' — the prevention or termination of problem individuals or groups," said Wess. "They favoured sterilization among the German population, as well as, of course, extermination for other specific population groups. Those we remember. But what was so quickly forgotten were the extensive experiments with genetic monitoring for selection purposes, especially in psychiatry." According to Wess, whole counties were registered, often without the knowledge of the people being monitored, and the records served as targeting devices for eugenic initiatives such as involuntary sterilization and euthanasia. "The careful, methodological, rational application of eugenic principles throughout society," Wess reiterated, "far from being aberrant or primitive or 'German,' in fact expressed the views and values of contemporary international genetic science itself."

People we associate today with the most grotesque, brutal, and apparently nonsensical experimentation were also part of this effort. Dr. Josef Mengele, the infamous Auschwitz doctor, collected biological specimens in the concentration camp under the direct supervision of the internationally known geneticist Otmar von Verschuer, his former teacher and scientific superior, and sent them to Verschuer for his work in genetics at the Kaiser Wilhelm Institute for Anthropology,

Human Heredity and Eugenics in Berlin. Verschuer burned the evidence of his association with Mengele after the war, though Wess claims Verschuer's past was an open secret in scientific circles. Verschuer went on to become a leading figure in genetics in the 1950s, heading the German delegation to the landmark first International Conference on Human Genetics in 1957, and he trained German geneticists until he died in the 1960s.

One of the major international figures of the eugenics of the thirties was Frederick Osborn, a scientist at the Carnegie Institute and later at the Rockefeller Foundation, who preferred a eugenic society that was not enforced by the state. "Osborn said that eugenics could only work when we make the people think and act eugenically without noticing it," Wess explained. "He said one of the first points is to establish a society with a certain standard of living, a consumer society where you can buy everything, including health. Then we have to make the family smaller, so the parents will think about the quality of the life of their children. Then, with this consumer society of small families, people will start to think eugenically, because in such a society, success depends on performance — economic performance above all. This will be the real starting point for people beginning to choose what kind of children they will have, to act in a fully eugenic way."

For Ludger Wess, as for Udo Sierck, Heidrun Kaupen-Hass, and many other German critics, the real agenda of contemporary reproductive and genetic engineering is a eugenic one, a fulfillment of Osborn's vision. Wess's conclusions, which sounded extreme to my Canadian ears, are routine in Germany. "I think that a great deal of genetic research should just stop, or be stopped, altogether. Research on the genetics of 'intelligence' and certain kinds of 'mental illness' has no scientific basis in my opinion anyway. But I say this regardless of whether this research can give us some insight into the biological background of intelligence and mental illness or not. I think that these insights are very much outweighed by the negative social and political consequences for people. For me this extends to all the technologies of prenatal diagnosis, even the ones that have been accepted, because of the way they participate in the assessment of the quality of a life."

This evaluation is shared by many others, including the American-born, Hamburg-based molecular biologist Paula Bradish. Bradish served for three and a half years as scientific adviser to the Greens in Bonn in the mid-eighties, when a German parliamentary commission on the risks of genetic engineering was preparing its report. She is now involved in studying the biological and social implications of various genetic technologies, specializing in industrial food production and processing (and currently doing work on human genetics as well). In a café across the street from the offices of the Hamburg Institute for Social Research, a non-profit foundation where she now works, Bradish spoke bluntly. "Genetic engineering from humans through animals and plants right down to microorganisms is eugenic because it's about deciding which gene is more or less useful, more or less valuable." She's convinced the basic principle behind both reproductive and genetic engineering underlies much of modern science. This is the notion "that nature is something that is mechanistic, that it can be improved upon and that it actually must be improved upon; that living beings of all kinds are, if not actually defective, at least in need of repair, of being made more efficient."

For Bradish, the central question is the same as for Ludger Wess and Udo Sierck: who decides what is more "useful?" "While contemporary eugenics may not be dictated from above by the political programs of dictatorial regimes," she says, "the pressures of the market are as forceful and destructive, if not more forceful and destructive, than what we have had in the past." The NRTs are being offered by individual doctors to individual women; there is no state or formal coercion. But the "private" decisions made by women and their doctors nevertheless reflect what kind of life is privileged and welcomed in the social and economic arrangements of our society — what kind of child is a "wanted" child. "The selection of genes according to their evident usefulness is the same," says Bradish, "whether we're talking about bacteria or human beings."

The social danger here is that by practising these technologies on ourselves we will treat humans more and more in the same mechanical way we treat plants and livestock — which can pose major problems in human rights. In fact, through the impersonal and seemingly apolitical functions of the marketplace, contemporary pressures to abort potentially disabled or female fetuses (female being a category of economic disability in some societies) are close to Frederick Osborn's vision of eugenics-without-knowing-it.

The second danger is physical. As various disasters in the creation of transgenic organisms (organisms with genes from two species) have unfolded with regularity — as pigs given human growth hormone, for example, developed arthritis, or potatoes created for their "chipping" qualities turned out to be poisonous, or hybrids bred to combine the vigour of African bees with the honey-collecting dedication of European bees emerged from a laboratory in Brazil in the 1970s as lazy, destructive killers — the record of spectacular failures presents a fundamental challenge to the dominant genetic theory.

This is the record to which the molecular biologist and virologist Regine Kollek, a colleague of Paula Bradish's, has been pointing in her scientific attack on the theory and practice of genetic engineering. Her field is risk assessment in microbe, animal and human genetic engineering. "Animals are very complicated systems," Kollek explained. "What we see when new genes are introduced into the embryos of animals is that this process cannot be completely controlled. The development of animals is so complex the introduction of new genes often disturbs these finely tuned processes. And what we see is on the one side with animals, they grow faster with lower fat, which is essentially the goal of the experiments. But on the other side, they become far less stable in terms of their whole health condition." In other words, and this is no mean trade-off, we may experience a net loss, not a net gain, from genetic intervention.

In her publications, Kollek has attacked the science of genetic engineering in terms of its understanding of the nature and function of the gene itself. For her, as for a number of dissenting scientists internationally, current practices in genetic engineering derive from a simplistic and incorrect evaluation of how genes work. "There is a great deal of evidence that says that the gene is not an isolated, self-contained 'blueprint' that can be moved about from cell to cell or tissue to tissue or species to species," said Kollek. "How genes act depends not only on what information they 'contain' but also on their location in the cell and their relationship to other genes, on their context as well as their content." It is the relationship that is meaningful, not the isolation of one component. "Above all, the recombining of genes produces what we call 'emergent' properties," said Kollek.

"These are new properties, which by definition cannot be predicted. The current paradigm is blind to these dimensions, and therefore potentially very dangerous."

In the United States, as well as in Europe, many transgenic microorganisms already have been released into the environment for purposes as diverse as preventing frost on strawberries to consuming oil spills in the oceans, without long-term consideration of their eventual impact on the whole ecosystem. In 1988, the United States government quietly opened up a bureau to monitor such consequences, and such a bureau has recently been established in Great Britain, too. But at the same time, by funding massive genetic research, notably the Human Genome Project to map the human chromosomal picture at Lawrence Livermore and Los Alamos laboratories, the U.S. government is richly sustaining the genetic paradigm Kollek criticizes. The Canadian government has recently awarded $17-million (matched by another $5-million from the National Cancer Institute) to a group of Canadian natural scientists to participate in the Canadian Genome Project.

Kollek-type objections to genetic engineering have been derided by mainstream scientists for many years, but several recent discoveries have suggested that she is on the right track. An article in the *New York Times* on February 6, 1992, reported on the finding of the gene for myotonic (muscular) dystrophy, which affects one in 8,000 babies born today. What was simultaneously discovered was that the gene gets worse from one generation to the next. This flies in the face of the "unchangeable blueprint" theory of genes on which genetic engineering is based. Dr. Bert Vogelstein, a molecular geneticist at Johns Hopkins University School of Medicine, "said that now that it has been established that a gene can grow and become more mutant with each generation, geneticists have to consider the startling possibility that other mutant genes might gradually cure themselves over generations."

In the March, 1993, issue of *Scientific American,* John Rennie reported a series of further discoveries with "heretical" implications in a lengthy article called "DNA's New Twists": "Contrary to expectations, genes sometimes leap from one chromosome to another, or expand and contract like accordions. Chromosomes seem to carry chemical tags that identify whether they originated in an organism's mother or its father.... Workers have even found indications that organisms may be able to respond to changes in the environment by altering their genes."

Rennie tellingly quotes researchers discovering the keys to a remodelled view of genetics — for instance, Jeffrey W. Pollard, a developmental biologist at Albert Einstein College of Medicine: "DNA isn't this inert thing encased in Lucite, sending out instructions. It's part of the cell, and it's responding to what's happening around it."

Such discoveries add weight to Kollek's stern warning that we will pay a high price for intervening in processes that we do not yet fully understand. But Paula Bradish says that this intervention is likely to proceed, regardless of the new evidence, because the investment of billions of dollars in the biotechnologies in recent years has created an economic momentum that, in the absence of social resistance and political action, will be unstoppable.

The new *reproductive* technologies — pharmaceutical ovulation-induction, sperm and egg manipulations, surgical insemination, Petri-dish fertilization, embryo transfer, embryo banking, and the like — are concerned with the creation of a human embryo. *Genetic* technologies, on the other hand, are concerned with the embyro's quality. The cluster of new reproductive techniques, however, are handmaids to the genetic technologies, for without them the human embryo would not be open to judgment and genetic manipulation.

Today, in London, Ontario, Jeffrey Nisker, a reproductive endocrinologist and in-vitro fertilization specialist, is performing pre-implantation diagnosis aimed at screening out embryos with a genetic predisposition to severe mental retardation. First, an eight-cell embryo is created in a Petri dish, then two of its cells are extracted for biopsy and examined for signs of the predisposition. Then the embryo-minus-the-quarter-of-its-original-matter is implanted in its "mother's" uterus or rejected on the basis of the findings of the biopsy. In England, where this technique was pioneered, success rates for embryo survival are staggeringly low — which never seems to stop anybody.

In the genetic field, there are three major sub-clusters of technologies: prenatal diagnosis, such as amniocentesis and chorionic villus sampling, in which genetic material is analyzed to permit genetic abortion; "somatic" intervention, in which genetic material is introduced into a subject to effect a therapeutic goal in that individual alone, as in some projected treatments of Parkinson disease,

Huntington disease, Alzheimer's, and diabetes; and "germ-line" genetic intervention, through which all succeeding generations emanating from the individual will also be affected. Pre-implantation diagnosis is critical to this last.

Critics of genetic engineering have warned for years that germ-line intervention is the logical and inevitable extension of genetic research. Leading genetic researchers have belittled and dismissed their fears, denounced them as paranoid and extremist, and claimed that germ-line manipulation should never be, would never be, undertaken in humans. But the fears of the critics are being borne out. In August, 1991, Mary Warnock, medical philosopher, head of the Warnock Commission, which set the fundamental direction for British policy on the new technologies in the mid-1980s, informed a press conference that germ-line manipulation "needs enormously more caution, but simply to say we should never do it is to be short-sighted." With these qualified and seemingly innocuous words, the first official step over the genetic Rubicon was taken. Two months later, for the first time, the National Institutes of Health subcommittee on human gene therapy considered at its Washington meeting techniques for genetic manipulation of human eggs. Industry (Nikon, for example) has already developed a way to mass-produce the electronic micromanipulators involved in pre-implantation diagnosis, and markets them aggressively at international conferences and symposia worldwide.

In Germany, the Embryo Protection Law, passed in the summer of 1990, prohibits the creation of human embryos for research purposes and other forms of genetic experimentation on embryos. (Nevertheless, when embryos are created during IVF, often not all embryos are implanted in the women, leaving "surplus" embryos, as they are known, in embryo banks around the world.) In Britain, by contrast, the 1990 Human Fertilization and Embryology Act has given the green light to pre-implantation diagnosis and approved the use of human embryos for research.

Because procreation takes place inside women's bodies, women are the living sites of intervention for reproductive and genetic engineering. In Germany, as elsewhere, feminists have been the most active organizers against the unquestioned proliferation of the technologies. Many women have become radicalized by their encounter with the practice of reproductive medicine, on the one hand, and the feminist movement on the other. For instance, IVF and infertility specialists have played up their pregnancy success rates and downplayed side effects of the technologies. Feminist critics, along with German natural and social scientists, were among the first to point to a variety of serious hazards posed to women by the high-dosage "hormonal cocktails" involved in medically-assisted procreation, suggesting the likelihood of long-term problems for the women as well as pointing out dangers for the IVF babies themselves. Such critics are now being joined by other medical and epidemiological specialists, as evidence begins to mount on the hazards. A recent ovarian cancer study indicates a twenty-seven times increase in ovarian cancer among women who have taken fertility drugs but who did not become pregnant. (There was a two-fold increase among women who did become pregnant.)

One of the most important German centres for feminist activists can be found in a draughty old brick-and-stucco building at the back of an obscure courtyard off a nondescript street in the industrial city of Essen. The Gene Archive, presided over by a dedicated group of women health professionals and activists, collects everything it can find through its national network on reproductive and genetic engineering. Its major emphasis is on humans, but it also maintains files on agricultural and other applications. (A major archive and organizing centre for agricultural and environmental applications, the Genetic Network, is funded by, among others, the Green party, and is based in Berlin.) The Gene Archive, which shares office space with the medical practice of Dr. Beate Zimmermann, serves not only as a focal point for many women activists in Germany, but as an important resource base for the Feminist International Network on Reproductive and Genetic Engineering, a loosely associated web of women's groups and individuals involved in similar issues all over the world.

A number of German feminists had been working on reproductive and genetic technologies since the late 1970s. But the big feminist surge that spread grass-roots women's groups throughout the country took off from a conference of more than 2,000 women, including feminist critics from the U.S. and many developing countries, held in Bonn in 1985. Organizations termed "direct action" or "terrorist" also took up the cause — in 1987 raiding several genetic laboratories, taking research records, and making them public. One research centre was bombed.

According to Ulla Penselin, who served time in jail for aiding a "terrorist organization," the militant actions gathered a lot of support. "Though many did not see these actions as means they would personally employ," she explained, "the feeling in many parts of the women's movement and beyond was 'It's not my way, but if some women want to do this, okay.' " The group that aroused the most sympathy was Rote Zora (Red Zora), which was, according to Penselin, "a cell of women not living underground, but doing clandestine actions."

Because of the importance of the biotechnology and pharmaceutical industries to the German economy, the growth of this opposition caused great consternation in both government and industry circles. Parliamentary commissions were struck to investigate aspects of the technologies and heated political debates ensued between the various protagonists. Until the militant actions of 1987, the discourse had been confined to words. Then all hell broke loose.

Dr. Beate Zimmermann recalled how just before Christmas in 1987, "things were quiet at the Gene Archive. Two of my patients were sitting in my waiting room down the hall, when all of a sudden all these policemen came crashing through the door with riot equipment and machine guns. They took everything, every scrap of paper. They destroyed things, and they took me to the station, where they were very rough with me and did a strip search. Of course, there was absolutely nothing else they could do with me after that. The whole thing was preposterous."

Preposterous, but serious. At the same moment the police were busting the Gene Archive in Essen, they were conducting more than twenty other raids on people connected with feminist services and groups across the country. In the end, of all the women brought in for questioning and arrested, only Ulla Penselin and another woman served prison terms.

"The German government used that excuse to attempt to criminalize the whole movement, to intimidate us, to frighten us into silence," sociologist Ute Winkler told me as she fielded telephone calls requesting information on women's reproductive health matters at the Frankfurt Feminist Women's Health Centre. "And, no question about it, there was a lot of fear at the beginning. But in the end, the whole thing actually backfired because a huge public-defence campaign was launched that included many different religious and political groups. We were not successful in freeing the two women. But we were able to further raise awareness and opposition to reproductive and genetic engineering. It has been a very tough fight."

Their opponents are not unique to Germany: multinational pharmaceutical companies, scientists and research institutes, both public and private, supported by a plethora of smaller entrepreneurial biotech businesses, and an emerging layer of medical fertility specialists ("technodocs" as they like to refer to themselves) and genetic technicians dominate and shape the field. The expanding markets in North America, Europe and, increasingly, among the upper classes of the Third World, are in proceptive (profertility) technologies; in Asia, Africa and Latin America, and among the lower classes of the First World, they're for contraceptive (antifertility) technologies. (The German women's movement has done more organizing than most other First-World women's movements against the notorious use of Third-World women as guinea pigs for contraceptive drugs and technologies not permitted for testing at home.)

The medical industries involved in reproductive and genetic medicine are also looking towards sensational market expansion and profitability in the coming decade. Speaking at the 6th World Congress of In Vitro Fertilization and Alternative Assisted Reproduction in Jerusalem in 1989, IVF specialist Dr. Bernard Lunenfeld estimated that at that time the potential market in the industrialized world for fertility drugs alone amounted to 10 million women, joined every year thereafter by an additional 700,000. (One cycle of fertility drugs can cost up to $2,000, not including IVF. Women routinely do three cycles, six cycles are frequent, and ten not unusual, with or without in-vitro fertilization.) The profits from these and other drugs and procedures are staggering.

Some pharmaceutical corporations are direct or indirect owners of IVF clinics, including major research centres such as Bourn Hall in England, where Patrick Steptoe, "techno-father" to Louise Brown, officially the first "test tube baby," presided until his death in 1988. Ares-Serono, the largest manufacturer of ovulation-inducing drugs, heavily subsidizes many international conferences and symposia for physicians and nurses, technicians and scientists. Through its nonprofit educational branch, Serono Symposia, it also helps fund infertile couples' networks such as

Resolve Inc., the largest infertile couples' support organization in the U.S. Serono was on hand in 1990 in Ottawa when a group of Canadians set up a similar organization (funded to the tune of $500,000 by the Tory government in the same year that government axed funding to feminist services across the country), and simultaneously opened up their Canadian subsidiary. Other corporations, such as Bristol-Myers Squibb at Toronto's Mount Sinai Hospital, fund genetic research on animals (mice in this case) with the understanding that the corporation may have right of first refusal for commercial applications. But because no central registry of reproductive and genetic research and development exists, it is difficult to know the full extent not only of the research itself but of the connections between commercial and noncommercial elements. (NAC's brief to the Royal Commission has asked that such a registry be established immediately in Canada.)

The Montreal sociologist and former Royal Commission member, Dr. Louise Vandelac (she and three other commissioners were fired by Brian Mulroney in 1991), calls the development and proliferation of reproductive and genetic engineering a manifestation of "science-push" (or "the technological imperative"). Scientists, often funded by the pharmaceutical corporations, develop a given technology, and industry then aggressively markets it through a largely unregulated medical system. The press duly announces another medical miracle, the technology is institutionalized with a legion of medical personnel, who then develop their own economic stake in the technologies, and presto! a whole new norm for pregnancy is established. (Ultrasound prenatal diagnosis is now used in more than eighty-five percent of Canadian pregnancies. One former cabinet minister told me that she was treated "like a social traitor" by a specialist when she refused to have an amnio for her "high-risk" pregnancy at the age of thirty-eight.)

The term "techno-industrial imperative" might be more accurate to describe the dynamic. But whatever one calls it, the process preempts any public discussion; the market and the medical systems usurp what should be a fully democratic process.

In Berlin, I spoke with Dr. Gertrud Gumlich, an internist and a member of the Supreme Synod of the Protestant Church (roughly equivalent to our own United Church), about the church's criticisms of the new technologies. Gumlich explained: "From our point of view, just because something is possible in medicine or technology does not mean we should do it." To a large extent, church views are based in a traditional religious evaluation of the sacredness of human life and the importance of the bonds of relationship and responsibility in procreation. As far as genetic selection is concerned, as in most matters of life and death, the church is happy to leave it to (a divinely motivated) nature, strongly confirmed in its position by the hideous and hubristic experience of the Third Reich.

Many of the questions the church has raised, however, particularly about the commodification of human life, overlap those of the secular, academic critics. "We have major questions about the ensuing problems for children, parents and science too," said Gumlich. "These are ethical questions. What does it mean, for example, to have this new category of potential human life, the so-called 'surplus' embryo? What does it mean to make experiments on this embryo? We don't like abortion, but we do not say women who abort are criminals. They do it under terrible pressures because they feel they must. But with these technologies, we are voluntarily taking positions on larger social choices about our attitude to human life, and the church is asking hard questions about them." Submissions made by certain church representatives to the Canadian Royal Commission during its public hearings in 1990 echoed these concerns. But in Canada, as in the U.S., Catholic opposition dominates, and it is fundamentally based on a commitment to denying women abortion, making feminist/church collaboration difficult here, at least to date.

The German feminist sociologist Ute Winkler stressed the importance of real public debate and making common cause. "Yes, it is important to fight for laws as we have done, but what must ultimately count is the development of alternatives and simply a refusal by women and men to use the technologies. Because laws can be overturned." Indeed, all the German laws stand to be overturned if the European Parliament harmonizes the laws in the European Community on reproductive and genetic engineering. "Because most countries do not have laws like the ones we have in Germany," Winkler said with a tired sigh, "we will lose the good work we have done here."

As we await the report of our own Royal Commission on New Reproductive Technologies, I ask myself once again: to what extent are the Germans clear-sighted as a result of their historical experience? To what extent are the technologies bearers of destructive values? Are there indeed ways in which some of the technologies can be helpful? To what extent can we think of them — or some of them — as neutral, their effects dependent on who controls their use, as their most progressive proponents argue?

Even before my trip to Germany, I believed that Canada should place existing IVF programs under research rather than treatment protocols, with the attendant cautions and restrictions demanded when research is being done on human subjects. I was convinced that the technologies related to in-vitro fertilization were a bad idea, with extremely low success rates, enormous costs and a variety of serious known and projected physical and social risks to women and children. With the new findings on health risks coming in, I have come to think that we should stop allowing this procedure to be offered. I don't believe IVF can be made a healthy, safe or effective technology, even if women were to control it (as Utopian a notion as slowing down proliferation of the technology long enough to have a proper social debate). As an infertile woman who lost her fertility to a previous reproductive technology (the Dalkon Shield) I am deeply aware of the terrible pain that can be associated with infertility. I simply think that the physical risks to both women and children are too high.

As far as the eugenic dynamic of the new genetic technologies now offered through prenatal diagnosis is concerned, I have tended to share the views of McGill geneticist and epidemiologist Dr. Abby Lippman, who is also chair of the Human Genetics Committee of the Council for Responsible Genetics in the U.S. In the March, 1989, issue of *Current Therapy,* Lippman wrote, "We cannot only celebrate the opportunity [genetic screening] may provide individual women to make personal decisions about being tested and about selectively aborting fetuses. We cannot only condemn the eugenic possibilities inherent in the use of prenatal diagnosis should public acceptance of the abortion of fetuses with serious disabilities be but the start of a slide down this particularly ugly slope.... Neither extreme pro or con position recognizes the political and social context in which testing occurs; neither addresses how either an individual woman or a public policy can or should balance or otherwise harmonize our often irreconcilable and clearly incommensurate attitudes to women, to fetuses, to the medicalization of pregnancy and to disability." Lippman was arguing for developing an approach to these technologies that takes into account a multiplicity of realities, first and foremost those of women and children, and the social context of their lives, and to use this as our starting point for the evaluation of whether and how these technologies are deployed. What that means in concrete terms I, along with many other Canadians, am still struggling to figure out. Lippman, keeping company with other scientific and feminist critics, condemns embyro research and germ-line manipulations, and wishes to ban them.

My conversations with German critics — as well as what I have learned in Europe and North America about the enormous economic and social pressures now exerted on women to make genetic selections for potential disability and sex — have clarified for me the "ugly slope" that indeed exists, here and now. Even when the mechanism of eugenic selection is market-driven, it is a very powerful one — perhaps, as Paula Bradish warned, even more powerful than one imposed by the state because it wears the appearance of "choice."

Look around, and you see the new eugenics everywhere. When medical insurance companies begin to contest their obligation to provide medical coverage for babies carried to term despite an amniocentesis result that indicates disability; when governments compel doctors, as California now does, to offer pregnant women prenatal diagnosis; when children can win suits for "wrongful life" against parents who bore them knowing they had genetic anomalies; when private and public corporations become involved in genetic monitoring of employees: under such circumstances individual women can only conclude that they must, for their children's sake as much as their own, make genetic selections where they can. And "where they can" is an ever-expanding category, determined by commercially driven scientific research, with those terrible questions hanging over it. What criteria will we use to decide what life and what qualities are more worthy than others? Who will choose what life is worthy and for whom will they choose? And — the really scary one — who will control how worthy life is made?

When, as in France today — where the ratio of IVF cycles per woman is seven times greater than in the U.S. because of public-health funding of IVF procedures and a national mania for technology — healthy women in their early twenties are routinely arriving at IVF clinics asking them to "make a baby" after three months of unprotected intercourse; when leading IVF doctors suggest that all embryos should be subjected to pre-implantation diagnosis as a step towards family well-being and public health; when, as in Canada and the U.S. today, pregnant women are being held in custody, kept artificially alive or operated on against their will in the name of their fetuses' rights; when international teams of doctors and scientists are developing techniques to mature ova from female fetuses and cadavers; when genetic sex selection is being used around the world to allow for the abortion of unwanted female fetuses: when all these developments are taken together, it seems clear that some combined version of *Brave New World* and *The Handmaid's Tale* is already taking shape within our own society.

These are extremely powerful technologies. Their impact has been compared by many responsible and erudite natural scientists to that of nuclear technology. Either we gain control of their development and deployment in a conscious social fashion, or their proliferation will create de facto changes in reproductive relations and social values, whether we like it or not. Though each technology needs to be evaluated in terms of its own risks for each individual and family, the main dangers lie at the collective level — for women as a group, for society as a whole, for future generations — as a result of the cumulative impact of these technologies on our reproductive lives.

German opponents of the new technologies are calling for a halt to further proliferation, and for a diversion of economic and social resources into dealing with the social causes and consequences of infertility and disability. The World Health Organization has also called for a moratorium on the creation of new IVF facilities, until much more accurate evaluations can be made of the extent and options for infertility. Marsden Wagner, former director of the Copenhagen-based Department of Maternal and Child Health for the World Health Organization, estimates that for every IVF baby born, thirty cases of infertility could be prevented.

It has also been estimated that more women become infertile every month in the United States as a result of pelvic inflammatory disease than have successfully had babies through IVF worldwide since it became available in 1978. Nevertheless, Canadian governments spent $3.5-million in 1987 on new reproductive technologies research, while only $400,000 went into public-health services research and health research related to reproductive disorders.

In Germany critics have raised fundamental questions about the new reproductive and genetic technologies from a multitude of perspectives. The recurring consistency and moral authority of their views, centred around the core issue of the "new eugenics," argues that at the very least we carefully consider their conclusions before we proceed any further. They are suggesting that when it comes to reproduction and health, what helps with plants and animals also helps with people. The principles of variety, multiplicity, complexity and co-evolution are what must finally guide our relation to nature, including the nature within us. These, they suggest, are what must replace the ultimately totalitarian impulse to dominate, control and reshape nature that continues to guide most reproductive and genetic research today.

The long-awaited report of our Royal Commission is likely to sanction continued proliferation, rather than recommend a slow-down or a halt. Even though a study of Canadian fertility programs prepared for the Royal Commission was highly critical of IVF clinic practices, claims of success, record-keeping, patient follow-up, and aspects of safety especially related to the risk of AIDS from the use of fresh sperm, Patricia Baird's public reaction focused on how to rectify the failings rather than on the tenability and safety of IVF itself. Given the severity of the potential consequences of these technologies as measured against their limited gains, the cautionary words of the German critics are crucial to heed. We are not ready — scientifically or socially — for artificial intervention into reproductive and genetic life. Let us stop — or at least seriously slow — the train of proliferation, before we find that, though we do not want to arrive at its final destination, we cannot get off.

PART III

THE ROYAL COMMISSION ON NEW REPRODUCTIVE TECHNOLOGIES: A COSTLY FAILURE?

The Royal Commission was a major investment for Canada in terms of finances ($25,000,000), personnel and effort on the part of many. Although the final report has not been released at the time of writing — it has already been delayed three times — the manner in which the Commission has conducted its business has been a deep disappointment for many Canadians.

This section looks at some of the things that went wrong: Christine Massey describes the flawed public participation process; Margrit Eichler details the internal structure of the Commission and critiques the research process; and the Statement of Claim by four ex-Commissioners remains an unhappy monument to a process that became derailed. Louise Vandelac puts the operation of the Commission into a broader economic and political context, and suggests some reasons why the commission went the way it did.

When this book was begun, we hoped people who had worked for the Royal Commission would write of their experiences. This was a greater demand than we anticipated and anonymous contributions from six former researchers for the Commission detail why they were afraid to come forward with signed statements, or be more explicit in their descriptions of what went on.

When we read these anonymous statements, we wondered whether we had stumbled upon the sole disgruntled exceptions or whether these statements were typical for many — though certainly not all — researchers for the Commission. Consequently, midway through this project, we sent a questionnaire with just two questions to everyone who was listed in the Commission's *Update* of August 1992 as having done work as a researcher for the Commission. We asked: "Is the attached listing correct? (If not, please correct here.)" and "How would you describe your experience with the Commission?"

We received 148 replies. These varied from one word responses ("excellent," "positive," "negative") to a sentence or two, or a paragraph or two, to long, detailed letters. With regard to their listing, 76 of the respondents corrected one or another aspect. Some were minor (misspelling of a name, an incorrect affiliation, professional title, degree or paper title), while others were more substantial and included people who — though listed — informed us that they did not do any work for the Commission (true in 6 cases).

Not all respondents provided a meaningful answer to the second question. Some simply stated "I did..." without commenting on the quality of the interaction, but several responded with qualitative details. Of these, 69 indicated that the experience had been positive, while 37 — about one third — said that it had been mixed or negative, with responses here ranging from complaints about unrealistic timelines to expressions such as it "was a nightmare."

We make no claims about the "scientific" nature of this brief survey and hope that readers will put these responses into the context of the papers in this section in forming their own assessment of the failure of the Royal Commission.

12

FRANKENSTEIN MEETS KAFKA: THE ROYAL COMMISSION ON NEW REPRODUCTIVE TECHNOLOGIES

Margrit Eichler

There are two metaphors which crop up repeatedly when people who had dealings with the Royal Commission talk about it: one is that it was a Kafkaesque situation, the other, that there was a Nixonian cover-up and obfuscation. For instance, one former researcher writes: "The closest parallel I can think of to the atmosphere of suspicion... is the White House during Nixon's cover-up."[1] A journalist describes his dealings with the Commission as "Nixonian in obfuscation."[2] Another former researcher writes: "From the outset, the conventional medical model of research prevailed, augmented with a rigid hierarchical structure. Frankenstein meets Kafka."[3] The ex-Commissioner Louise Vandelac repeatedly describes the Commission as "Kafkaesque." Yet another journalist uses the same word to describe the Commission dealings.[4] In this article, I will attempt to trace the development of this situation and reflect on what it means for the Commission's final report.

The Commission was created in October 1989, with an initial reporting date of October 31, 1991, later to be changed, first, to October 1992, then to July 1993, and finally to November 1993.

The Commission was set up as the result of a two-year, large-scale, intensive lobby effort[6] of the Canadian Coalition for a Royal Commission on New Reproductive Technologies — a nation-wide coalition of women's groups, health groups, other groups and many individuals.[6] In April 1989, the federal government announced in its Throne Speech as the main thrust of its social policy for that session that a Royal Commission would be created.

It took until October 1989 for the Commission to be launched, with one of the broadest mandates of any country. The original Order-in-Council charged the seven appointed Commissioners:

> ... to inquire into and report on current and potential medical and scientific developments related to new reproductive technologies, considering in particular their social, ethical, health, research, legal and economic implications and their public interest, recommending what policies and safeguards should be applied...[7]

Dr. Patricia Baird, a paediatrician and geneticist in Vancouver, was appointed Chair of the Commission. The other Commissioners included: Dr. C. Bruce Hatfield, a private practitioner in internal medicine in Calgary; Martin Hébert, a member of the law firm Guy and Gilbert in Montreal; Dr. Grace Marion Jantzen, a lecturer of Religion in London, England; Maureen McTeer, a lawyer from Ottawa; Suzanne Rozell Scorsone, director of the Office of the Catholic Family Life Archdiocese of Toronto; and Dr. Louise Vandelac, a professor of sociology from Montreal.[8] The mandate obliged the seven Commissioners to jointly engage in the actions that would enable them to report their findings to the government.

From the outset, there were extremely serious problems, although few of them were publicly visible at the beginning. The major ones can be identified as follows:

* an undemocratic internal structure was established by the Chair, which prevented Commissioners from participating meaningfully in discharging their duties and which resulted in anomic staff relations;

* a manipulative public participation process was instituted which gave the appearance of public participation while precluding genuine participation on the part of many;

* the research process was cloaked in secrecy and rigidly controlled. The Chair treated the research as her unilateral responsibility, rather than that of the Commission as a whole — while failing to maintain the normal standards of Canadian social science research.

The overall picture that emerges is one of a Commission tightly controlled by one individual — the Chair — who was determined, against all opposition, to carry through her personal game plan. This was made possible by a federal government which went to extreme lengths to back up the Chair and her autocratic decision-making at crucial times when serious challenges were posed.

In the following, I shall examine the internal structure and the research process. I omit a discussion of the public participation process, since this matter is dealt with in Massey's paper in this volume.

INTERNAL PROBLEMS

From the very beginning, problems as to how the Commission was run were noted by the majority of the Commissioners. The problems concern such issues as the conduct of internal Commission meetings,[9] the nature and timing of public participation, the content, timing and location of Commission meetings,[10] the overall goals and framework for the Commission's work, the time allocated to various matters[11] and above all, the research process. Commissioners wrote numerous letters and memos with proposals and requests that were repeatedly ignored or outright rejected. In particular, several Commissioners asked repeatedly for *in camera* meetings, i.e., meetings just among the Commissioners, without staff present, to discuss these management problems. The Chair consistently refused to hold such meetings. They later summarized the experience as follows:

> ... *from the very first meeting, the collegiality hoped for has not materialized. Instead, any attempts at collegiality have been continually undermined and over time it became apparent... that all substantive decisions about every aspect of the Commission's work were being made under the authority of one person, namely the Chairperson, Patricia Baird.*[12]

Examples of the exclusion of Commissioners from the work of the Commission abound. For instance, the Commission conducted a public opinion poll which had serious methodological flaws. The Commissioners, pointing this out, received a promise that the poll results were for internal use only, and would not be released to the public. Nonetheless, they discovered through press reports that the results had been released.[13]

Similarly, they learned from a communication from the Director of Research that the Chair was expecting an extension of the reporting date, which meant that she must have previously requested the same without consulting the Commissioners.[14]

In another instance, a new round of public consultations was scheduled in 1991 against the written dissent of the majority of Commissioners (Hatfield, Hébert, Knoppers, McTeer and Vandelac).[15]

In the same vein, the report "What we heard: Issues and Questions raised during the public hearings" was released as an official Commission document against the strongly expressed disagreement of four of the Commissioners. Hatfield, Vandelac, Hébert and McTeer wrote to Baird to inform her that they had discussed the paper and

> write to advise you that under no circumstances will we agree to this publication. The concept, purpose and content of this letter and "document" are fundamentally flawed. No amount of tinkering will render it acceptable as a paper, from this Commission, to be sent to thousands of Canadians and the press.[16]

The document was released anyway.[17]

After having exhausted all other avenues to persuade the Chair to adopt a more democratic leadership style, including making repeated requests orally and in writing and finally boycotting meetings, four of the seven Commissioners — Hatfield, Hébert, McTeer, and Vandelac — requested a meeting with the Clerk of the Privy Council, in the presence of the Chair, to resolve the differences and clarify and confirm professional and democratic working relations among Commissioners. In their letter, they informed the Clerk, Mr. Paul Tellier, that the majority of Commissioners (four of the seven) had stopped attending meetings, thus depriving the Commission of a quorum. They defended their actions stating that the Commission's manner of conducting its business "makes a mockery of the most basic rules of democratic functioning," leading to a pervasive ineffectiveness, and to the incapacity of the Commissioners to discharge their functions in an appropriate manner. The Commissioners therefore asked for "an intervention from the highest political and administrative levels" to resolve the impasse.[18]

This meeting eventually took place in August 1990. Although expected to attend, the Chair sent word at the last minute that she would not come. The Clerk of the Privy Council noted, in agreeing to a meeting, that "commissions of inquiry stand, or fall, independently from the Government."[19] Notwithstanding this statement, shortly after the meeting, the government appointed two more Commissioners — Bartha Marie Knoppers and Susan McCutcheon — and changed the original Order-in-Council so as to grant exclusive decision-making authority to the Chair. Although Commissioners were thus deprived of their rights under the Public Inquiries Act, they remained responsible for producing a final report on the several issues raised by the Commission's mandate.[20]

The government's unusual decision to appoint two additional Commissioners so late in the life of the Commission[21] effectively disempowered the original majority. No change in the exclusive rule by the Chair has been noted. Further, the unexpected and unprecedented change of the Order-in-Council — unique in the history of Royal Commissions in Canada — saw the federal government actively interfering with the internal workings of a Royal Commission in a manner profoundly consequential for the outcome of its work (the final report). The purpose of Royal Commissions of Inquiry has always been to put the discussion and research of issues of importance to society beyond the political realm. The government's actions — still unexplained and undefended today — effectively frustrated meaningful research and genuine public discussion of the issues raised by science and medicine's new-found ability to create, manipulate and alter human life in the laboratory, by retroactively legitimating the undemocratic actions of the Chair.

Neither the meeting with the Clerk of the Privy Council, nor the change in the original Order-in-Council, resolved the issues at stake. If anything, relationships and processes within the Commission worsened. They centered around various issues, but the one which demonstrates most clearly the Kafkaesque situation created by the Chair concerns confidentiality.

In the fall of 1990, three of the Commissioners fluent in French gave press interviews to the French language press, at the latter's request. During these interviews, they raised their concerns about the fair and open operation of the Commission and their frustration at being excluded from all key decisions and work of their mandate. When asked, Commissioner McTeer had to admit that she knew nothing about the Commission's total budget. *Le Soleil*[22] and *Le Journal de Québec*[23] ran articles quoting the Commissioners.

The day after, at the next Commission meeting (which was the first with many Research Directors), Susan McCutcheon, one of the two new Commissioners, raised the issue of the media interview in the context of a breach of the Commission's confidentiality. The three Commissioners so accused, namely Vandelac, McTeer and Hébert, requested an *in camera* meeting to discuss the issues raised. The Chair refused to entertain their request, but allowed other Commissioners to continue the discussion and accusations. Scorsone, for instance, suggested that the interviews were "a personal attack which could be personally damaging to Patricia [Baird]. Perhaps it isn't too bizarre to wonder whether it might qualify as defamatory libel under the Criminal Code."[24] Outraged at being falsely accused of criminal action, Commissioners Hébert and McTeer protested, demanding that the matter be adjourned to an *in camera* meeting of Commissioners before any further issues were discussed. Again the Chair refused, but declared that the issues, having been raised, would now be left unresolved while matters of research were discussed.

Subsequent to this meeting, the Chair unilaterally sought — at public expense — a legal opinion with respect to confidentiality within Royal Commissions. Baird later informed the Commissioners of this in writing:

I am, as Chair, formally requesting you... to refrain from any further public discussion, whether in the press or elsewhere, of the internal, confidential discussions of the Commission, including matters relating to its management....

I would like you to provide the Commission... with a statement of your receipt and understanding of the policy laid out above and your intention to refrain from any further public discussion of the internal activities of the Commission..."[25]

She refused, though, to substantiate the claims of criminal wrongdoing by certain Commissioners or to provide them with a copy of the legal opinion. Here is where things got truly bizarre. All Commissioners indicated — reluctantly — in some form or other, that they accepted the principle of confidentiality. However, the falsely accused Commissioners denied that there ever was a breach of confidentiality on their part. Baird cited the legal opinion obtained by her, but refused to send it to the accused Commissioners, since they had not yet satisfied her personal demand to sign her confidentiality pledge in a manner which she found acceptable. In the end, a threat of legal action against her forced her to release the opinion from the former federal Deputy Minister of Justice, then in private practise in Toronto. The opinion had little to do with the issue at stake and did not find any possible action under the Criminal Code against the accused Commissioners.

Eventually, the Chair accepted all the pledges of confidentiality except the one made by Vandelac. Deeply perplexed, Vandelac copied verbatim the pledge made by Hébert, which Baird had accepted from him as satisfactory.[26] In receipt of Vandelac's letter, Baird replied: "The statement made by Martin Hébert is perfectly acceptable, for Martin Hébert."[27] She continued to refuse to accept Vandelac's promise not to breach confidentiality. Instead, she required once more that Vandelac sign a special pledge that she would send to her. In the meantime, Vandelac would be prevented from attending meetings and participating in the Commission's work. At a meeting held in Victoria later that fall, the Chair sought to exclude Vandelac. Having failed to do so because of the solidarity of three other Commissioners, she cancelled the Commission's meeting. Finally, a compromise was struck. Baird had half the Commissioners meet with the research staff in the morning and the other half in the afternoon.[28]

As the attempts at exclusion continued, Vandelac, in desperation, retained a lawyer with extensive experience in Royal Commissions. He wrote to Baird.[29] Oddly, soon after this letter was sent, Baird found, upon reading one of Vandelac's previously mailed letters, that she had, indeed, pledged confidentiality in a manner which Baird now said was satisfactory to her.

All of these things were happening while the public hearings were going on — hardly a situation which would facilitate a genuine exchange of opinion between Commissioners and those members of the public who were presenting their briefs to the Commission.

Matters did not improve after the famous pledges of confidentiality were signed. In some ways, the time which some Commissioners were required to devote to staving off false accusations concerning confidentiality effectively denied them the opportunity to shape the substance and content of the all-important research program. Commissioners were consistently unable to find out what research was being undertaken under the Commission's aegis. The information provided to them was all but meaningless, although it was presented as being comprehensive. Projects were approved, disapproved, initiated or altered by staff under the sole direction of the Chair. All comments provided by Commissioners were requested after the projects had been approved by the Chair. As such, their comments and work served no purpose but to allow the Chair to say publicly that Commissioners had been consulted on the research program.

On December 6, 1991, four Commissioners took the unprecedented action of filing a suit against the Chair and the federal government, in which they sought to overturn the second Order-in-Council as contrary to the Public Inquiries Act. They sought guidance in the neutral forum of the Court on how to resolve this intractable problem and asked that if their claim was sound that they be granted sufficient human, technical and financial resources to enable them to discharge their duties.[30]

Exactly ten days later, on December 16, when Parliament had adjourned for the Christmas recess, they were fired.[31] As one columnist stated: [It was a] "Machiavellian move: it's now unclear whether the four have any legal standing in their own lawsuit."[32] One of the dismissed Commissioners, Hébert, "accused the government of firing the four to block a court fight over the issue of the revised mandate that could have gone against the government."[33]

Having been fired, the four ex-Commissioners lost their standing before the federal Court, and were obliged to drop their suit. The matter of the legality of the second Order-in-Council, and thus the Royal Commission itself, remains unresolved and the Canadian public remains largely unaware of these crucial events surrounding the Commission's activities and use of millions of public funds.

THE RESEARCH PROCESS

Although there were multiple serious problems within the Commission, none was as important as that involving the research program — which one would assume would be the backbone of the Commission's final report.

It was not only Commissioners who were unhappy. One of the former staff recalls the "reign of terror which governed the workplace arousing paranoia and distrust in many of us and eroding our sense of solidarity and commitment."[34] Another writes "Walking past that building in Ottawa still makes peoples' hearts pound, because they remember that fear."[35] Yet another stated "... people involved with the Commission were labelled, laid off and silenced and... ideas were manipulated, distorted and embellished in order to ensure a certain result."[36] Finally, another one said that "Dissent from the dominant discourse was not tolerated at the Royal Commission, and it was always punished. Dissenters were marginalized, and their activities monitored. Surviving became a full time occupation."[37]

We received these comments (which are published in this volume) from former researchers and staff under the condition that we would keep their names confidential. In order to find out whether these comments were representative of others, we decided to send a one-page questionnaire to all "researchers"[38] listed in the Update of August 1992. We asked two simple questions: "Is the attached listing correct? (If not please correct here.)" and "How would you describe your experience with the Commission?" We had a good response[39] and obtained some interesting results. Out of the total of 148 replies, 76 made a correction in their listing. Of these, six stated that they did not do any work for the Commission.

Fifty-five percent of the respondents found errors in their listing — a troubling rate.[40] Equally troublesome is the possibility that this may be indicative of the care with which the documents were prepared. It should be noted that this report was issued after the majority of the research staff had been fired.

Some of those who replied to our questionnaire were highly complimentary of the Commission. Their comments ranged from one word statements to separately attached letters which extolled the virtues of the Commission. However, 37 of the replies were either completely negative or a mix of positive and negative. (Forty other replies were without a qualitative component and have not been classified as either positive, negative or mixed. This includes the six respondents who reported that they had not done any work for the Commission.)[41] Some of the negative statements rivalled those received from our anonymous contributors. For instance, "My working relationship with the Royal Commission on New Reproductive Technologies was a nightmare." The reply goes on to list the details. Another lengthy reply states, "My experience... was totally frustrating." One reply, which came in the form of a 4 1/2 page single-spaced typed anonymous letter states:

> *My time at the RCNRT was an exercise in futility, frustration, and disillusionment. In my view, the manner in which the Commission was conducted was a betrayal of the Commission's staff, researchers, Canadian women in general, and feminists in particular.... my departure came with my realization that continued association with the Commission would make me complicit in the perpetuation of an anti-woman policy making process...*

Another reply which was sent in anonymously (with the listing cut off) sums up by stating that "in my opinion, the Commission was a disaster mainly because of upper level management's incompetence and the desire to ram through a pre-set agenda."

The reasons for other negative comments are varied, but they include unrealistic deadlines, lack of feedback and vague instructions. This, however, must be balanced against the replies of other people who laud the Commission staff, often naming one or two specific individuals who are identified as particularly helpful, professional or responsive. Many drew a clear distinction between "the Commission" (the Commissioners) and the staff, whom they characterized as helpful, professional and competent.

The most troubling responses were those which suggest that an attempt was made to shape the nature of the findings. It is this aspect that I shall attempt to examine here.

The Chair hired an Executive Director (John Sinclair) and a Director of Communications and Coordinations (Dann Michols) almost immediately following the establishment of the Royal Commission, but delayed the appointment of a Research Director until early summer 1990.[42] This delay is quite extraordinary. Arguably, the single most important function of the Commission, integral to the writing of its final report, is its research program. It is because they felt such a strong need for original, first-hand research that Coalition members had fought so long and hard for the Commission to be established. Yet even with an unlimited public budget, the Chair took one third of the Commission's entire initial mandate to hire a Research Director.

It is even more remarkable that a research structure, dividing its researchers into four "task forces," was put into place by the Chair and the Executive Director, prior to hiring a Research Director.[43] The Commission finally hired Dr. Susan Mann, then Vice-Rector, Academic, of the University of Ottawa. She resigned after three weeks.

The Chair thereupon found and hired a new Research Director, Sylvia Gold. However, in the summer of 1992, in response to the firing of almost all of the research staff, she too resigned. In June 1990, four of the Commissioners — the majority at that time — having come up against numerous difficulties including several unsuccessful attempts to discuss the research process, wrote a letter to Dr. Baird, informing her that they would no longer participate in meetings until their concerns were adequately addressed: "... There remained an almost complete lack of public awareness of this Commission's existence; no comprehensive communications and consultations strategy; and, most important of all, no research program.... [A] limiting and undemocratic structure... [has been] imposed upon us..."[44] Dr. Baird replied:

> ...My reading of the situation is that this Royal Commission has accomplished a great deal... As Chairperson... I have consistently sought consensus on all matters pertaining to the work of the Commission.... I would ask you to reconsider your position...[45]

This preceded the meeting with the Clerk of the Privy Council and the swift change in mandate and addition of two Commissioners referred to above. The concerns that led the Commissioners to request the meeting were reiterated by Maureen McTeer in a letter to Dr. Baird:

> ...the research component of our work has been seriously (some would argue irretrievably) undermined. Eight months into our mandate, we have been advised in writing that a Research Director has been hired. Yet there is no research plan and no possibility for a full discussion of what research needs to be done and by whom, prior to the fall. [46]

Hatfield, Martin and Vandelac endorsed McTeer's letter: "... that a single person, and a geneticist to boot, would be responsible for such a dossier, would no doubt be considered as a flagrant lack of objectivity and deep conflict of interest..."[47]

About a year later, the Commissioners were still trying to determine the nature of the Commission's research. At a Commission meeting in June 1991 in Halifax, which four of the Commissioners were unable to attend, research was apparently discussed. Two information sessions were set up for the four who had missed the meeting — one in July for Jantzen, another in August for Hébert, McTeer and Vandelac.[48] The latter meeting was a somewhat stormy one and for good reason. Two years after the Commission began its work, it was still refusing to provide Commissioners with a complete and comprehensive research plan including:

* titles and numbers of all the projects of the four working groups;
* timetables (dates of contracts granted, project start-ups and interim and final reports);
* names of researchers;
* budgets allocated;
* initial research specifications prepared by the internal teams, including project objectives, their relevance to the Commission's work, methodologies, etc.;
* comments by all Commissioners.

Furthermore, we were surprised to say the least that Research and Evaluation then claimed we had received all these documents. [49]

"Extremely annoyed,"[50] the Commissioners then drafted a memo requesting the detailed work plan, a progress report on projects and all initial research proposals, including those revised and those rejected as well as those accepted with reasons why they were rejected.

> If we are unable to obtain this basic information, we will be entitled to wonder about the significance of all this pseudo-consultation concerning the research projects, which clearly appear to have been contracted out despite our strongest reservations, and indeed our fiercest opposition. If the term "consultation" merely means being able to claim that the Commissioners have been consulted, our personal and professional integrity is clearly at stake....[51]

As a result of this effort, the Commissioners obtained a listing of research projects, containing neither names of researchers, nor budgets, timetables or project descriptions. Nevertheless, "from the project titles and numbers, we were able to deduce the extent of the research program and to see that, for some sub-groups, we had got wind of only five of more than 30 projects."[52]

Most of the Commissioners criticized this inadequate listing of projects.

Baird confirmed her denial of the requests made by the four Commissioners in a memo she addressed to all Commissioners:

> Some Commissioners have requested changes to the Commission practise with regard to receiving information on research contract budgets and on the identification of research contractors....
>
> After weighing the pros and cons of identifying individual contractors, I remain convinced that providing such information is not the best policy for the Commission....
>
> I have also reviewed the question of providing budget information for each project. As I stated in Calgary, using dollar figures as an indication of the importance or priority of any given project is not appropriate and is misleading for a number of reasons. It is difficult to compare dollar figures between contracts simply because the cost structures vary so much, with different per diem rates being charged by contractors (which often reflect regional and professional factors), the time the contractors invest, and different overhead costs being assessed by host institutions. This latter, for example, may range from 0 percent to 65 percent of the cost of the project. In addition, there is a significant cost difference between secondary analysis and primary research but these cost differences do not reflect their relative importance or impact regarding the formulation of our recommendations....[53]

It is truly extraordinary that the refusal to provide budget information was phrased in terms of potential misinterpretations of these figures. The Chair obviously considered herself capable of adequately judging the relationship between dollars expended and the importance of a project. If, indeed, the other Commissioners lacked the mental competence to do the same, one would expect that this could be explained to them in the same terms as the above-quoted memo.

However, Baird did promise the Commissioners "an integrated project listing of *all* research activities in one document."[54] The Director of Research, at the request of the Chair, sent a memo to the Commissioners explaining how to read the summary sheets on the various research proposals, called project arrays. The project array consisted of pages with four columns: "Project Number and Title," "Current Status," "Manuscript to Commissioner for Review" and a blank column headed "Commissioner's Notes." As an overview of research this was virtually useless. It provided none of the details as to what any of the projects entailed. The Commissioners concluded:

> ... Commissioners have been provided with so little information that they have no knowledge of more than half the research program....
>
> Only the Chairperson, together with some research and evaluation staff, has been able to analyze, change, approve and reject projects, thus shaping the entire research program from fall 1990 to winter 1991.
>
> This proposal review process is thus completely devoid of all meaning... [it] appears to support the illusion that Commissioners are taking an active part in developing the research program and that a true multi-disciplinary effort is ongoing, when in fact the information we are given is partial, we are excluded from the entire decision-making process, and the proposals are not even discussed collectively.
>
> ... any claim that the Commission is making a serious effort to review research proposals is ridiculous...."[55]

By accident, the Commissioners obtained through non-official channels the work plans for the Commission's research for all four working groups.[56] These work plans contained all the information repeatedly requested by the Commissioners. It also showed that the research projects which Commissioners were asked to comment upon during the summer of 1991 had already been approved in January of that year by the Chair, acting alone. Research staff realized this, but the Commissioners, acting in good faith, did not. As set out in the Statement of Claim, the entire research program was directed and approved by a person who, as a geneticist, is both judge and jury in determining public policy on one of the most important series of issues to confront Canadians in this century.

A former staff member comments on how this affected the work atmosphere at the Commission:

> ... the unconfirmed and speculative nature of the information... contributed to a climate of suspicion and paranoia at the Commission. During November and December 1991, shortly before the four 'renegade' Commissioners were fired, staff members were virtually paralyzed. Staff members were aware of rumours that the firings were imminent, yet there was no information as to when the firings would occur, and what impact this would have on the Commission's future operation.[57]

This person goes on to recall having a conversation with one of the Commissioners who was eventually fired, and then being interrogated by the supervisor about the nature of the conversation.

> While it was never stated outright, the implicit message was that staff had no right to communicate directly with the very people they had been hired to serve, Commissioners. Staff were instructed... to complete 'record of phone conversation' forms every time we spoke with a Commissioner. It was understood by staff that these forms were a way of spying on Commissioners.[58]

On December 6, 1991, the Commissioners filed their suit and ten days later they were fired. The only reason offered by the government for this unprecedented action was the need for the Chair to finish her report on time. Since then, she has requested two additional extensions to November, 1993.

After the firings, there were rounds of public protests and repeated calls for the resignation of the Chair and the reinstatement of the four Commissioners, all of which were ignored.[59] The Coalition re-established itself and wrote to the Prime Minister asking that he

> 1. disband the Royal Commission on New Reproductive Technologies immediately;
>
> 2. have all research projects evaluated in an independent review process;
>
> 3. make appropriate monies available through an alternative mechanism to conduct the necessary research;[60] and
>
> 4. proclaim a moratorium both on any expansion of existing or an initiation of new infertility and genetic services...[61]

A month later, the Deputy Clerk, Security and Intelligence, and Counsel, replied to the Coalition's letter to the Prime Minister of January 29.

The Commissioners were selected for their demonstrated abilities to deal effectively with the complex and sensitive issues within the Commission's mandate. Like other commissions, this Royal Commission has been given the independence to determine what, in its opinion, are the best methods for dealing with the issues confronting them.[62]

Early in 1992, mounting concern about the continued secrecy surrounding the Commission's research, (which after all is funded by tax monies and was set up in response to citizens' requests for research), prompted the Social Science Federation of Canada (representing 15,000 Canadian social scientists), to establish a task force charged with examining this matter. This group made repeated attempts to obtain adequate information from the Commission. These included: repeated letters from the President of SSFC to the Chair of the Commission, requesting information about the research program,[63] and a meeting with Commission staff[64] at which the requested information was promised, and repeated follow-up letters when it was not forthcoming. In June 1992, the President of the SSFC stated in a letter to Dr. Baird, "your response is clearly unsatisfactory"[65] and reiterated the request for a written response to the issues identified. He announced that if there was no adequate response the Federation intended to "combat what is turning out to be your Commission's blatant disregard to the norms of research."[66]

Left without an adequate reply, the President of SSFC wrote to the Prime Minister in July 1992, detailing its attempts to obtain basic information concerning the Commission's research. "We have now waited over two months for this basic procedural information, but to no avail.... your Government has invested 25 million dollars of the taxpayers' money in a Royal Commission which is refusing to provide basic information to Canadians about the research it is undertaking.... We urge you to intervene immediately..."[67]

SSFC's requests for information were strikingly similar to those made earlier by the fired commissioners, and others.[68] But once again, their efforts were in vain.

In July 1992, the President of the Canadian Association of University Teachers (representing all 60,000 professors in Canada), wrote to Dr. Baird stating "... we are astonished at the secrecy which you are maintaining concerning the individual researchers and their projects."[69]

Some time later, Baird replied to the letter of the SSFC President of June 12, 1992: "The Commission is pleased that so much interest has been shown in our programs and how we have gone about our task...." and enclosed with her letter a copy of the August 92 *Update* which provided a listing of individual researchers by name and nature of involvement.[70] It was in this publication (used as a basis for our one-page questionnaire described above) that we found a 50 percent inaccuracy with respect to the listing of those who responded.

The *Update* contained the following description of the Research Process:

> *Research proposals were solicited and reviewed by Commissioners and external peer reviewers for content and methodology. Researchers' names and institutions were not identified, as Commissioners felt this would help promote greater objectivity on the part of those reviewing proposals and enable them to evaluate the material on the merits of the content....*
>
> *Once a project was completed and a manuscript received, it too was reviewed by both Commissioners and external peer reviewers. The authors' names remained confidential until after this review had been completed.[71]*

These assertions are false. Four Commissioners felt themselves compelled to begin a law suit in Federal Court to obtain information about research proposals and reports. They had argued consistently that secrecy about researchers would not "help promote greater objectivity" — indeed, quite the contrary. The Chair's response not only speaks to the credibility of the research program, it also speaks to the issue of honesty. The public has a right to know how and for what purpose public funds are being spent. They also have a right to be told the truth.

The Social Science Federation of Canada reviewed the material and noted:

> *... despite its promise to do so, the Commission has not provided descriptions of the research projects, without which it is impossible to assess what research is being done, and how it is being conducted. In addition, the details of the peer review process and solicitation process are insufficient to determine whether the Commission has followed the usual procedures of scientific inquiry.*

They characterized what has occurred as a "highly irregular research process"[72] in a further letter to Baird, to which she replied,

Commissioners are pleased with your continuing interest in our work. We regret, however, that the Federation finds the information we have furnished at the meeting in April and the subsequent newsletter insufficient. We have worked hard to put the issues, and information on them, before Canadians....[73]

In November 1992, the Commission announced that it had sought and obtained another extension of its mandate to July 15, 1993.[74] In June 1993, the reporting date of the Commission was changed for the third time, this time to November 1993. This new date pushed the release of the final report beyond the expected federal election and removed the issue from the likelihood of public discussion during the election campaign process.

DISCUSSION

Hynes[75] has drawn a parallel between how the atomic bomb was developed and how biotechnology in agriculture in the U.S. is being introduced. Unfortunately, the model she presents may provide some clues towards understanding what has been happening with NRGTs and the Royal Commission in Canada. Hynes identifies several crucial factors including:

* *A mythology encases the technology to make it necessary and acceptable. Once it becomes technically possible, it becomes inevitable.*
* *Regulation and policy are used to protect the technology, to ensure that it can profitably survive conflict, public distrust, and even failure....*
* *The new technology is not presented as one among many solutions to a problem, but as the dominant one. The alternatives to the technology are shut out.*[76]

If one intended to make the NRGTs acceptable to the general Canadian public, it would make sense to go to extreme lengths to keep research under wraps, in defiance of the normal procedures and in the face of the opposition of the entire research community. It seems reasonable to speculate that the veil under which the research process was hidden means that there were issues that the Commission did not want to be publicly examined. Yet research programs must be judged not only on what is done, but also on how it is done, as well as on what is not done.

The hiding takes various forms, of which perhaps the most insidious is the recurrent tendency to respond to statements of critics merely by asserting that what has been challenged has already been done. This happens again and again.

For instance, just after the Commission was criticized for its lack of transparency in its research process, the failure to fully describe the peer review process and the failure to follow normal standards of research, it described its research process as follows:

> *[The Commission] is committed to an open and transparent research process. It is also committed to a process that adheres to the standards set by other quality research organizations.... Peer review for content and for methodology is a key feature in the process.*

After four Commissioners sued the Commission to find out what research projects were underway, and after having documented their lack of input at the proposal stage (as well as at all other stages), the Commission stated, "Research proposals were solicited and reviewed by Commissioners and external peer reviewers for content and methodology."

In the first Newsletter after the four Commissioners were fired, "A Letter from the Chairperson" stated:

> *In mid-December, I was informed that the federal government had revoked the appointments of four of the Commissioners. Over the past two years, I had worked hard to ensure that Commissioners had the opportunity to participate fully in all aspects of the Commission's work. I have encouraged, and will continue to encourage, full and open discussion of the issues.*

No word about the lawsuit, no word about the issues underlying it. Simply a global assertion of the Chair's openness to full participation on the part of all.

Critics who wrote to the Commission were blandly thanked for their interest in the Commission's work. A charge that it had shown "a blatant disrespect for scientific norms of research, including a transparent research process,"[77] elicited the Commission's reply: "Commissioners are pleased with your continuing interest in our work."[78]

The Coalition had decided in the first place to press for a Royal Commission, rather than some other type of investigatory panel, because of the broad powers that Royal Commissions have. Royal Commissioners "have the same power to enforce the attendance of witnesses and to compel them to give evidence as is vested in any court of record in civil cases.[79] Since it is notoriously difficult — as it should be — to obtain medical data, this seemed the appropriate mechanism to acquire the basic empirical information that would allow the Canadian public to judge the various reproductive and genetic techniques.

The powers and the budget — $25 million — of the Commission were sufficient to support and carry out the basic research that needed to be done.

As we cobble together the various scraps of information, a disturbing picture of their research emerges. Returning to the responses to our questionnaire, one person commented:

> *The research program could have been better designed and articulated and should have started much sooner than it did.*

Another person commented:

> *I did question to some extent the relative emphasis on review of existing evidence, which in some areas was lacking, vs. commissioning or support of original research, which, although time consuming could have added to the limited body of knowledge in some aspects of infertility.*

It is impossible to judge the extent to which basic research was, indeed, conducted (as opposed to preparatory steps including reviewing existing literature, applicable laws, reports and opinion polls). Yet, there are several indications that comparatively little effort was spent on the former and a disproportionate amount on the latter. The list supplied in *Update*, even given its inaccuracies, indicates a great emphasis on surveys, literature reviews and secondary data analyses. What is at issue here is not the adequacy of any individual study, but the adequacy of the total mix of all studies.

Another clue comes from several other comments elicited by our questionnaire.

One person detailed one of two involvements as follows:

> *I participated in the initial "Explorations Conference" where a number of people with different expertise from across the country were gathered to help the commission set its agenda and process. That was an especially bizarre experience where most participants I spoke with felt the name of the game was to keep us from actually developing ideas.*

Several respondents commented in detail upon the lack of depth in the research with respect to their specific areas:

It's unfortunate that health promotion and the primary prevention of reproductive disorders, which was regarded as a side issue, was not given greater prominence on the Commission's agenda... This is unfortunate, since preventive initiatives addressing the risk conditions that lead to reproductive disorders — STDs, socioeconomic inequities, workplace hazards, etc. — would go a long way towards reducing the demand for costly, suspect technological interventions.

Another commented:

In my own area, the level of research undertaken was extremely disappointing.

A person who reviewed two papers comments: "I suggested that the work be re-done, it was so thin."

Another person commented:

As many as one in five women have endometriosis. As many as one in three women with endometriosis is infertile.... It is my opinion that the Commission should have reported in more ways in which modern technology is now addressing endometriosis-related infertility.

Another person related:

Though I have been asked three times to collaborate with others on Royal Commission... projects, I have each time refused to do so. The reasons? I believe that this commission['s]... way of working merited little credibility...

The most disturbing types of comments we received had to do with possible attempts on the part of the Commission to shape the research findings. Here are some examples:

Our submission was initially returned with comments directing us to revise our paper in a manner that contradicted our primary thesis, so I wrote an eleven page response explaining why the requested revisions were unacceptable.

This person concluded with the comment:

Ours was the best experience with the Commission of anyone with whom I have discussed their Commission related activities.

Another individual wrote:

... my experience was definitely ambivalent.... The key word that kept coming back in our intital terms of reference and in subsequent comments was "balance." ...I got the strong sense that the Commission wanted a report that would address the medicalization charge levelled against NRTs and still leave the door open to further research and clinical application of them.

One researcher's comments were particularly interesting in that context. This person wrote:

I was instructed to limit my research to Canadian materials and to secondary sources. This prevented me from drawing on excellent secondary work on the U.K. and U.S. and created huge gaps where there were no Canadian secondary materials.

A person, (most likely the reviewer of the manuscript), commented in turn:

I provided a review of a research paper of which I was fairly critical. My main complaint was it was clearly commissioned work produced to speak to the narrow interests of Canadian doctors. I observed that most academics dealing with the subject would have felt less constrained and have drawn on American and European material. To my surprise I was telephoned and asked to defend my critique. Here again I felt, perhaps naively, that this was unusual.

A further clue is found in who is commissioned to do certain types of research. While the Commission did contract out research to many reputable scholars, it also made some choices in some crucial areas which are inexplicable if the intent was to generate an objective picture. The most drastic of these choices was the award of two contracts concerning the role of the pharmaceutical companies to Burson Marsteller — a public relations firm that represents pharmaceutical companies.

A former staff members sums up the situation as follows:

Researchers were viewed (by Patricia Baird) as an impediment to the drafting of the final report. It seems researchers were constantly irritating Dr. Baird by pointing out 'minor' problems, such as major gaps in the research.[80]

CONCLUSION

Kafka woke up one day to find himself metamorphosed into a giant cockroach. We are in the position of the horrified parents who find their child horrendously transformed. The Commission was set up in response to the efforts of many community groups and people. The Chair has betrayed these efforts in her systematic failure to conduct the Commission's business in a manner that would enable us to trust any recommendations that may be contained within the Baird Report.

ACKNOWLEDGMENT

I wish to thank Maureen McTeer and Louise Vandelac for a close reading of an earlier draft of this paper and their many suggestions for elaborations, and Lindsey Arnold for mailing out the questionnaire discussed in this article.

NOTES

1   See Anonymous #1 in this volume.

2   Stephen Strauss. "A scientific Cassandra recalls two future glimpses that went unheeded," *Globe and Mail*, July 11, 1992.

3   See Anonymous #5 in this volume.

4   Michele Landsberg, "Commission is crumbling under familiar Tory chaos," Toronto *Star*, January 11, 1992, p. H1.

5   This effort included, among other things, putting the coalition together, giving countless public speeches, meeting with large numbers of organizations, writing many letters to various politicians, meeting politicians, including various ministers, in their constituency or Ottawa offices, etc. Among other things, a meeting was held "on the hill" to bring the matter to the attention of politicians of all three parties. This meeting was attended, among others, by Marguerite Anderson, Martha P. Bielish, Patrick Boyer, Bob Brisco, Ed Broadbent, Pauline Browes, Pat Carney, Ethel Cochrane, Denise Cole, Mary Collins, Sheila Copps, Jennifer Cossit, Patricia Crofton, Marion Dewar, Joyce Fairburn, Sheila Finestone, Pauline Jewett, Don Johnston, Bob Kaplan. Others who were invited but unable to attend and who expressed their support included Bill Blaikie and David Crombie, while still others expressed their interest, including John Bosley and Bruce Halliday. Many of those who attended wrote afterwards in support of the Coalition to various Ministers.

6   The groups included: Alberta Advisory Council on Women's Issues, Alberta Status of Women Action Committee, Calgary Birth Control Association, Canadian Advisory Council on the Status of Women, Canadian Association for Research in Home Economics, Canadian Abortion Rights Action League, Centre des femmes de Verdun, DES Action/Canada, Gatekeeper's Project, Interaction Femmes-Santé, Inter Pares, L'R des centres de femmes du Québec, National Action Committee on the Status of Women, New Brunswick Advisory Council on the Status of Women, Northwest Territories Advisory Council on the Status of Women, Nova Scotia Advisory Council on the Status of Women, Ontario Advisory Committee on the Status of Women, Patients' Rights Association, Planned Parenthood Association of Edmonton, Planned Parenthood Federation of Canada, Planned Parenthood Ontario, Prince Edward Island Advisory Council on the Status of Women, Provincial Advisory Council on the Status of Women, Newfoundland and Labrador, Québec Conseil du statut de la femme, Regina Healthsharing Inc., Reproductive Alternatives Society, Reseau, Saint-Boniface, Saskatchewan Advisory Council on the Status of Women, Toronto Family Planning Network, Vancouver Women's Health Collective, Vanier Institute of the Family, Victoria Faulkner Women's Centre, Women's Inter-Church Council of Canada, Women Today.

7   See the Statement of Claim in this volume for the mandate.

8   *Ibid.*

9   Annex 1, dated April 1, 1990, of a working document to the Commission from Vandelac, appended to the memo by McTeer, Hatfield, Hébert and Vandelac to the Commission, of October 1, 1991.

10 E.g., four Commissioners vigorously protest against a unilateral announcement from the Chair that the next meeting of the Commission will take place in Vancouver — where the Chair resides — on September 5 and 6, 1990. As many staff members habitually attend these sessions, the Commissioners calculate that this choice of location will cost the Commission an extra $20,000. Much of this would be saved if the meeting was in Ottawa, since all staff are in Ottawa and several Commissioners are close to it. The choice of location is particularly surprising given that just five days later the Commission will again go west, to conduct hearings in the Yukon. Given that budgetary constraints are often cited to justify the feeble interventions with regard to the prevention of infertility and sterility, such expenses are even harder to understand. Summary of a letter by Hatfield, McTeer, Hébert and Vandelac to Baird, August 27, 1990. They state: "With this letter, we wish to dissociate ourselves clearly and unambiguously from such exorbitant and useless expenditure of funds, and we wish to communicate to you our most profound disagreement with this inconsiderate use of public monies."

11 E.g., in a letter by Hébert to Dann M. Michols, May 29, 1990, Hébert responds to a request by the Director, Consultations and Coordinations, for comments on documents that are slated for publication. He expresses his surprise at the speed with which these comments are required. The Commission used several months to agree on the wording of internal documents, but paradoxically, they are given 72 hours, namely one weekend, to provide reactions about documents which are about to be made public.

12 From the Statement of Claim, par. 13.

13 Letter from Vandelac to Baird, October 10, 1990.

14 Letter from Maureen McTeer to Pat Baird, Dec. 13, 1990, also the English translation of a letter from Hébert to Baird, January 8, 1991.

15 By the time this occurred, two more Commissioners had been added to the original seven (see below). Memo from Bartha Knoppers to all Commissioners, August 3, 1991; letter from Vandelac to Michols, August 9, 1991; memo from Bruce Hatfield and Maureen McTeer to Dann Michols, August 12, 1991; memo from Hatfield, Vandelac, Hébert and McTeer to Baird, August 14, 1991.

16 Letter from Hatfield, Vandelac, Hébert and McTeer, August 22, 1991.

17 Statement of Claim, paragraph 53, and Press release accompanying the document, Sept. 9, 1991.

18 Letter from Martin Hébert, Louise Vandelac, Bruce Hatfield and Maureen McTeer to Paul Tellier, June 26, 1990. The letter is in French, the quotes are translated by M.E.

19 Letter from Paul M. Tellier to Maureen McTeer, July 13, 1990. Translated by M.E.

20 P.C. 1990-1801 (from the Minutes of a meeting of the Committee of the Privy Council).

21 At that time, the final official reporting date was still October 1991.

22 "Le rapport sur les nouvelles techniques de reproduction risque d'etre 'tablette'," Le Soleil, August 27, 1990, p. A10. Translated by M.E.

23 Marc-François Bernier. "Mecontentement au sein de la commission royale," Le Journal de Quebec, September 27, 1990.

24 From the transcript of the 12th meeting of the Commissioners on Sept. 27, 1990.

25 Letter from Dr. Baird to Dr. Vandelac, Oct. 19, 1990, as well as similarly worded letter to McTeer.

26 Letter from Dr. Vandelac to Dr. Baird, Nov. 6, 1990, from English the translation in the Statement of Claim.

27 Letter from Baird to Vandelac, Nov. 14, 1990.

28 Footnote 2 of the English translation of a memo by McTeer, Hébert and Vandelac to Baird, Oct. 21 to Nov. 11, 1991. The French original dates this event as the end of November 1990, the English translation says 1991. Since the date on the English translation makes no sense, I have treated it as a typo and used the date from the French original.

29 Letter from John I. Laskin to Dr. Baird.

30 See the Statement of Claim, reprinted in this volume.

31 Geoffrey York and Ross Howard. "Dissidents fired from commission on reproduction," *Globe and Mail*, Dec. 17, 1991.

32 Michele Landsberg. "Commission is crumbling under familiar Tory chaos," Toronto *Star*, January 11, 1992, p. H1.

33 York and Howard, op. cit.

34 Anonymous #5.

35 Anonymous #1.

36 Anonymous #3.

37 Anonymous #2.

38 Many of them were, in fact, not acting in a research capacity, but as reviewers, consultants, participants in various colloquia, and other such varied capacities. The list of "researchers" provided is thus hugely inflated.

39 Of the 312 people listed, we could not find the addresses for 50. All in all, 262 questionnaires were sent out. Of these 24 were returned as undeliverable. Therefore 238 questionnaires presumably reached their addressees. We received 148 replies. This translates into a 62 percent response rate, a good result.

40 This was calculated as follows: Of a total of 146 responses, 7 replies were unclear. Deducting them leaves a total of 139. Of these, 76 respondents made a correction of some type.

41 This includes replies on behalf of people who had died, those who had, in fact, not participated in the Commission's work, as well as a number who wrote a short sentence "I did so and so" without a qualitative statement.

42 The candidates, who include Margrit Eichler, Abby Lippman, and Ralph Matthew, are told that there are four candidates.

43 The materials sent to one of the candidates, who was invited to apply, contain a write-up which outlines the decisions which have already been taken. "... the Chairperson and Executive Director of the Commission have designed the organization that will best meet and implement that mandate." It also notes obliquely that "The research and evaluation program has been the object of considerable discussion amongst Commissioners."

The package contains a description of the division of the research and evaluation branch into four task forces which had already been put into place. (From the recruitment folder handed to one of the candidates (Margrit Eichler), a sheet entitled Royal Commission on New Reproductive Technologies. The Research and Evaluation Program. Dated April 12, 1990. Emphasis added.)

44 Letter by Dr. Bruce Hatfield, Maureen A. McTeer, Dr. Louise Vandelac, and Martin Hébert to Dr. Baird, June 21, 1990.

45 Letter from Dr. Patricia Baird to Maureen McTeer, June 21, 1990.

46 From a letter by Maureen McTeer to Dr. Baird, with copy to Paul Tellier, June 28, 1990.

47 Letter by Dr. Louise Vandelac, Maitre Martin Hébert and Dr. Bruce Hatfield to Dr. Pat Baird, June 29, 1990, with copy to Paul Tellier.

48 The date is contained in the Sept. 4, 1991 memo from McTeer, Hébert and Vandelac.

49 From the English translation of the memo sent by McTeer, Hébert and Vandelac to Baird, Oct. 21-Nov. 11, 1991, emphasis added.

50 From the English translation of the memo sent by McTeer, Hébert and Vandelac to Baird, Oct. 21-Nov. 11, 1991.

51 Follow-up to meeting between Research Branch, Royal Commission on New Reproductive Technologies (Sylvia Gold, Director, Research, and four Research Coordinators), and Commissioners Maureen McTeer, Martin Hébert and Louise Vandelac, August 28, 1991, in Ottawa.

52 From the English translation of the memo sent by McTeer, Hébert and Vandelac to Baird, Oct. 21-Nov. 11, 1991.

53 Undated memo by Baird to all Commissioners, dated by fax machine as Oct. 15, 1991.

54 Undated memo by Baird to all Commissioners, dated by fax machine as Oct. 15, 1991.

55 From the English translation of the memo sent by McTeer, Hébert and Vandelac to Baird, Oct. 21-Nov. 11, 1991, emphasis added.

56 From the Statement of Claim, par. 46.

57 From the anonymous letter received in reply to our questionnaire.

58 Ibid.

59 Statement by NAC re "Dismissal of member[s] of the Royal Commission on New Reproductive Technologies, Dec. 16, 1991."

The Coalition, NAC, la Federation des Femmes du Québec, la Federation du Québec pour le Planning des Naissances, le Collectif de Sept Iles pour la Santé des Femmes, the Women's Health Interaction Collective, the Provincial Advisory Council on the Status of Women Newfoundland and Labrador, le Regroupement des Centres de Santé des Femmes, Naissance Renaissance, the Canadian Association for Women in Science [see Press release of the Canadian Coalition for a Royal Commission on New Reproductive Technologies, February 3, 1992] and L'R des Centres de Femmes du Québec [Telegram to Coalition, January 30, 1992] call for the four demands outlined in the January 29 Coalition letter to the Prime Minister.

The President of the Canadian Labour Congress writes to the Prime Minister, asking him "to immediately disband the Royal Commission on New Reproductive Technologies and to launch a parliamentary enquiry into the operation of the Commission." [Letter by Shirley G.E. Carr to the Prime Minister, February 10, 1992.]

The President of the Federation du Québec pour le planning des naissances writes to Dr. Baird in a widely circulated open letter to inform her that due to the problems in democratic functioning and the firing of the four Commissioners, "la commission a perdu à nos yeux toute credibilité et toute legitimité." [Letter by Anne St-Cerny to Dr. Baird, February 12, 1992.]

60 They have the Social Sciences and Humanities Research Council in mind.

61 Letter by Dr. Margrit Eichler to the Prime Minister, January 29, 1992.

62 Letter by W.P.D. Elcock to Dr. Margrit Eichler, March 2, 1992.

63 Letters by Dr. Robert A. Stebbins to Dr. Baird, March 13, 1992; April 8, May 7, June 2, 1992.

64 Letter by Dr. Robert A. Stebbins to Dr. Baird, April 8, 1992.

65 See letters from Baird to Stebbins, May 7, 1992; afterwards August 29, and September 29, 1992.

66 Letter by Dr. Robert A. Stebbins to Dr. Baird, June 22, 1992.

67 Letter by Dr. Robert A. Stebbins to the Prime Minister, June 19, 1992.

68 See, for instance, the description of Stephen Strauss of his dealings with the Commission which exactly parallel those of SSFC (and those of the four fired Commissioners):

    I asked the commission for names and proposals, and was told that getting this information would be physically impossible or at least very difficult. Besides, I was told, giving out the information would prejudice the science the commission's researchers were embarking on.

    Frankly, I didn't understand how this could be.... The whole process could be transparent; just tell us who is doing what and why they are doing it....

    A while later, a guide describing the commission's research was published which to my mind was positively Nixonian in its obfuscation. It contained no specific information about who was doing what research. It all but announced: Trust us, we're not crooks....

    The federation, like me, was stonewalled.... (Stephen Strauss. "A scientific Cassandra recalls two future glimpses that went unheeded," *Globe and Mail*, July 11, 1992).

    Other people had also been unsuccessful in finding out information about the Commission's research program.

69 Letter by Alan Andrews to Dr. Baird, July 21, 1992.

70 Letter from Baird to Stebbins, August 20, 1992.

71 Emphasis added, p. 3.

72 SSFC *Update*, Sept. 1992, Vol. 4 #4, 2nd p.

73 Letter from Baird to Stebbins, September 29, 1992.

74 *Update*, November 1992.

75 H. Patricia Hynes. "Biotechnology in Agriculture: An Analysis of Selected Technologies and Policy in the United States," *Reproductive and Genetic Engineering*, 1989, Vol. 2, #1, pp. 39-49.

76 Hynes, p. 40.

77 SSFC Update. April 1993, Vol. 5, #1.

78 Letter from Baird to Stebbins, September 29, 1992.

79 Inquiries Act, R.S., c.I-13, s. 1.

80 From the anonymous reply to our questionnaire.

13

INSIDE THE ROYAL COMMISSION

> *Anonymous*

ANONYMOUS 1

It is really hard to describe what it was like working for the Royal Commission on New Reproductive Technologies for two reasons. First, even over a year after my own work there ended, it is still very painful to think about the whole experience and second, it is almost impossible to explain exactly what was so terrible about it. Part of the problem was that so many of the people involved began with very high hopes that this was going to be a challenging and exciting opportunity to work with other intelligent and committed women on issues which were of particular concern to women. Instead it turned out to be the most destructive, competitive, unpleasant and overtly anti-feminist environment I have ever been exposed to.

It was particularly painful to watch some of the younger people who worked for the Commission, many of whom were very bright and committed feminists, first being astonished and disillusioned about what they saw going on, and then either leaving, or worse, staying and being co-opted into the power structure. For many this was their first "real" job and some were permanently damaged by the experience.

The real problem, far more serious than the division between the Commissioners which got so much publicity, was at the management level. To say that it was an example of "the Peter principle" in operation is putting it far too mildly. At the Director and Deputy Director level you had a group of fairly mediocre and wildly ambitious people (none of them feminists), most of whom were drawn from various backwaters in the federal government: fisheries, the Law Reform Commission, the Advisory Council on the Status of Women, the defunct Meech Lake team, or, worst, what is known in Ottawa as "the tank," the Management Centre, where unemployable civil servants with job security are warehoused until someone can come up with somewhere to ship them. From the first day these people saw and attempted to use the Commission as their route to a more prestigious job in the public service — in fact they all spent more time talking about what they hoped to do next (Assistant Deputy Minister was their most common objective) than doing any of the work at hand. The sort of questions which took up hours of management's time were who could fly first class, who could have free French lessons, and who was eligible to claim over-time. Many of these same people had also never handled staff before and they uniformly did it badly. The high turnover among the secretaries was just one indicator of the problem — these women recognized the place was crazy and got out. The Research Branch had almost as high a turnover; some outside researchers had their contracts handled by up to six separate staff members during the lifespan (about four months) of a single contract. Some of the Research staff who didn't leave (or get fired for being honest about something), went on thinking, naively, that they could somehow "fix" the place, or at least hunker down and do their own work well—neither turned out to be true. You really only realized how appalling the atmosphere was once you had left and were working somewhere normal again — without all the fear, conspiracies, in-fighting, etc.

Walking past that building in Ottawa still makes peoples' hearts pound, because they remember that fear: how the staff felt they couldn't be seen too often talking to the same people; how they were first told to always work with their doors open and then always to keep them closed; how the switchboard was told to monitor all incoming calls and report them to the "right" people who would then confront someone with why X was calling them; how when someone was fired no one dared talk about it and as the paranoia increased people would get back to their offices after being told they were fired (or "permitted" to resign) to find their computers shut down. The next day the combinations on all the locks would be changed — yet again. One night they even took down some walls looking for "bugs." The closest parallel I can think of to the atmosphere of suspicion all this created is the White House during Nixon's cover-up. While all this was going on it is not surprising how inefficient the Commission was and how little real work ever got done!

The only encouraging thing is that most of the people who played all the games and stayed the longest were ultimately often fired anyway—and many of them still haven't found jobs, so maybe there is some justice—but not enough. Some of the worst people are still there, earning big salaries, and dreaming of their next jobs. No one decent is proud of having been associated with the Commission; everyone I know just leaves it off their C.V. It was a terrible place to work.

ANONYMOUS 2

In response to the question "Why do I not feel I can write about my experience in working for the Royal Commission on New Reproductive Technologies," I have the following thoughts:

Talking or writing about the Royal Commission is prohibited by a clause in all contracts of employees and researchers on contract with the Royal Commission. The clauses in the contract state that we are not allowed to reveal information confidential to the Royal Commission, during the period of the contract or any time following. One might at first glance, as I did, think that the confidential information was of a substantive nature, perhaps research findings or the like. But it became clear that this was interpreted by the Commission to mean any information about the Royal Commission. Indeed, following the change in the order-in-council and the removal of Maureen McTeer, Louise Vandelac, Bruce Hatfield and Martin Hébert as Commissioners, the staff of the Royal Commission were asked to re-sign the "gag order" (as we came to call it). So legally, it is quite problematic to speak about what really went on there. The four Commissioners who tried to speak publicly about what happened were very quickly silenced. Given that these four people, with more status and influence than staff members, could be silenced with the full strength of the Federal Government, the message to the staff was clear; dissent is not allowed and will be dealt with aggressively.

I am therefore concerned about what could happen to me if I spoke about what really went on. It makes me feel incredibly frightened and vulnerable; so it is also that fear that keeps me from speaking. Generating fear was in itself a silencing strategy on the part of the Commission.

I think it is important that women in Canada who are working from a feminist perspective, whether in the area of the technologies or in any other area, understand that this gag order has to be signed by anyone who works for the federal government in any capacity. The intention behind the gag order is to protect the federal government and therefore the status quo. We need to critically assess whether or not Commissions called for by a federal government can ever achieve radical social change for women when powerful multinational corporations, such as the pharmaceutical and bio-technology industries in the case of this Royal Commission, are working to meet their own objectives.

Dissent from the dominant discourse was not tolerated at the Royal Commission, and it was always punished. Dissenters were marginalized, and their activities monitored. Surviving became a full-time occupation. Remembering the things that were done to and said about women, and feminists in particular, is very distressing and painful, which is another reason I am reluctant to discuss.

The final reason for my lack of willingness to talk about what went on there, is that when I have talked about it, it is clear that even close personal friends find it difficult to believe what went on. It seems incredible to them that these kinds of things happen, particularly in a democracy. Without understanding the full context, some of the things that went on seem ridiculous and silly. Without full disclosure, partial disclosure seems almost to trivialize what transpired there. The deep disappointment I felt in having had anything to do with a Royal Commission that treated people in the same way as the technologies treat women, as means to an end, will remain always. I am however much more aware of what is at stake for women if we do not collectively challenge the powerful technologies and the powerful institutions which seek to control our lives.

ANONYMOUS 3

The Royal Commission on New Repoductive Technologies is a difficult subject to speak or write about since the experience of many of us was one of profound disappointment and disillusionment. The reason that I have not come forward is because the experience was quite painful and remains so. It is also the kind of thing that no one would believe unless they lived it. Many started out with high hopes of exploring perhaps some of the most profound issues of our times from many perspectives and with an open mind. That this did not occur during the work of the Commission is perhaps not surprising. That people involved with the Commission were labelled, laid off and silenced and that ideas were manipulated, distorted and embellished in order to ensure a certain result is profoundly disturbing. I fear what has been compromised most by this Commission is the trust that women, in particular, placed in their hands to explore and report in a truthful, honest way about the impact new reproductive technologies will have on all of our lives.

ANONYMOUS 4

"On Doing Research for the Royal Commission on New Reproductive Technologies"

The process of social policy research is as important as the findings and outcome. It is therefore important to grasp the methodological crux of the matter, that feminist research is research for women, not on women. It is committed to improving women's lives.[1]

In the spring of 1991, I was invited to conduct research for the Royal Commission. At the time, the honour of doing a study for the Commission, which I considered to be an important inquiry, filled me with excitement beyond words. I had written to the Royal Commission expressing my interest in doing work in relation to its mandate, some time after the public hearing process was underway. But it was not until I had a conversation with another research consultant well connected to the Commission that an invitation was extended to me to conduct research for the Commission. Like a whirlwind, I was captured by the machinations

MISCONCEPTIONS: VOLUME ONE

of the Commission and official Ottawa. In a relatively short space of time, I was flown to Ottawa, where I met with staff of the Commission. I returned home to prepare a proposal, and within a matter of weeks, I received word to proceed with my study. Once ethics approval had been completed (which was, no doubt, expedited by the legitimacy of being Royal Commission-sponsored research), and the staff was hired, we got underway with a pilot and then the full study.

I began my study for the Commission with some trepidation. My reason was simple. From my earliest training as an undergraduate, I have been made to feel somewhat suspicious of contract research. As I passed through graduate school, and as I became ever more conscious of the close connection between consultants and powerful corporate (and state) interests, my suspicions about contract research intensified. I will always remember, in the summer of 1983, a woman employed by the tobacco lobby in the U.S. telling me that there was no solid research to support an association between tobacco and cancer, or at least none that adequately controlled for socioeconomic status. I remember thinking that this poor woman had been bought and paid for — exactly what I had always thought about contract researchers. The tobacco companies got what they had wanted — a skilled researcher who would tell them (and others) what they most wanted to hear. This example is replayed countless times, with researchers employed and/or funded by various corporate firms (e.g., pharmaceuticals, nuclear power, etc.) who have a product to sell to, or a need to contrive in, a very captive and fickle public.

So, imagine my surprise when I started my research for the Commission. They told me what they wanted (only the broad strokes of the study), and left it to me to identify the specific parameters of the study and the research protocol. I turned to the literature (including the feminist literature) as my guide, and explored what was known, what wasn't and carved out my own research objectives. Not a word was changed, nor an hypothesis altered in my proposal — nothing. I got a green light, and I was on my way.

The support I received from the Commission staff was wonderful. An able group of people were at my beck and call. Some staff changes created a glitch here and there, but nothing to cause worry. All in all, I hold those people in very high regard — the technical and professional staff at the Commission, who provided me with support.

So, for the first several months of my affiliation with the Commission, I would say the experience was not the least bit problematic. But before long, this picture seemed to change...

In the summer of 1992, things began to unravel. At first, I didn't pay events all that much attention. But as time passed, the unfolding of events consumed me. It began with the release of a *Research Update* that August by the Commission. The Commission had been challenged vigorously by the Social Science Federation of Canada to disclose how research contracts had been awarded (specifically the nature of the peer review process), and to whom. For reasons I am not privy to, the Commission remained tight-lipped. But then it released the *Update*, which provided a listing by discipline, by university, and then finally by research project. I checked to see that my project was listed and listed right. When I discovered that three other individuals were listed as co-investigators — neither of them known to me — I was more than a little disturbed! Who were these people? How did their names end up being attached to my study? A call to the Commission followed. I was told that many of the staff in the Research and Evaluation Program of the Commission had been laid off, and the Consultations and Communications Program staff had come in, gathered up files, and prepared the *Update*. A few mistakes had been found — not just by me. I chalked this up to carelessness, and considered it only a minor irritation. My concerns had been voiced. There seemed little likelihood that anything would be done about it, and besides, it would all come out in the *Final Report*, so what difference did it make? That was the end of that.

In the fall of 1992, I was sent my manuscript, along with comments from three external reviewers. One of the reviewers was highly complimentary, and raised relatively minor questions. The other two were brutal in their critique. When the comments were sent to me, I was told (verbally) that these were being sent for my information, and I was under no obligation to respond to the comments. (So why did they send them to me, I wondered?) I found some of the comments of the negative reviewers disturbing, not because the comments were critical, but rather because they seemed inappropriate. The reviewers' comments revealed their ignorance of social science. But never mind, I didn't need to attend to these criticisms.

In the winter of 1992-93, I once again received my manuscript from the Commission. I was asked to address some questions about my manuscript. This time, the questions came from "The Commission." As I started my way through the manuscript, I noticed that some changes had already been made to it by production staff, to clean up language and grammar. I recall coming to a statement in the manuscript, and thinking "wait a minute, I didn't write that!" and then concluding that nothing substantive had been changed. "They just cleaned up the language," I told myself. Then, the next query, and again, I thought "wait a minute, I didn't write that!" And this time, it seemed more than cosmetic. And again, and again. My thoughts turned to "wait one minute — this wasn't supposed to be how this turned out!" And the anger.

Then I got to a comment about my manuscript that sent me reeling. Why? Because there had been an attempt to alter what I intended to say, to tone down a point. "That's it! Out comes the original." And so, I sat there, going through the document word by word, page by page, making sure that my report said what I had said, not what someone far removed from the data and the research seemed to want it to say. I called the commission to seek clarification. I was told that I should make whatever changes I deemed appropriate. I was told they will be made, or if all else fails, I can pull my manuscript and it will not be published as part of the Commission's Final Report. And that's what I did. I prepared a lengthy, detailed letter asking that the text be restored. This has been done. And my study will be included in the Commission's Final Report. But this wasn't how it was supposed to be.

As I reflect on the research I did for the Commission, and the process involved in carrying out this type of contract research, there are at least a few troubling things that continue to resonate for me. First of all, although I felt privileged to conduct important (and I would add, feminist) research for the Commission, I felt betrayed when someone (an anonymous reviewer? a member of the Commission?) attempted to alter the substantive text of my report. To me, this was an infringement of my academic freedom. My frustration was compounded by the fact that, on balance, women who participated in my study generally spoke well of the services and service providers they had encountered. They had, too, spoken of their own conflicts and frustrations about accessing reproductive technologies. The person(s) who sought to alter the text could not see past, in my view, their own particular ideological agenda, and instead painted my report as overly ideological (obviously, the wrong kind of ideology!). Why, I continue to wonder, did they seek to make an essentially favourable report say things that the data would not support? What agenda was influencing the "review" process?

A second issue for me concerns what I see as an attempt to pervert my research findings. My research involved qualitative analysis in one section of the study. In my report, I prefaced the presentation of qualitative findings by saying that I would not cite the acutal number of women who had said this or that, but instead I would speak of "many," "some," and "a few" women who had said or experienced X or Y. In the review comments from the Commission (winter, 1992-93), I was asked to insert the number of women who had said X or Y. At one level, I would not have been troubled to report this (it would have been easy enough to go back to my coding sheets and analysis notes). But my sense was that the "reviewer" failed to grasp the essence of qualitative analysis, and was asking me to fit the women's narrative accounts into a quantitative mode. Meekosha describes this in terms of a need for "a spurious 'objectivity' through quantitative research."[2] I explained to staff at the Commission that when one does open-ended interviewing, information is sometimes volunteered that has not been specifically asked. If 5 women volunteer that they have had experience X, fine. This is reported, and accordingly validates the lived experiences of those individuals. If I am asked to report this as a proportion of the total sample, then these women's accounts run the risk of being trivialized, and the qualitative analysis is thereby corrupted. For argument's sake, suppose we have a sample 200, this translates to 2.5 percent of the sample. Reporting it this way misrepresents the data — it makes it seem that the other 195 did not have experience X. This was simply not the case. But this was what I was being asked to do.

As I look back on my experience with the Commission, I am still grateful for the opportunities that it provided me. However, I feel frustrated by the process of doing research for the Commission. I believed that my research would give women consumers an opportunity to be heard by the Commission. I hold steadfast to the belief that their voices were heard (even if there was an attempt to mute their voices somewhat). Yet, I am left wondering whether my research will be used, as Horowitz suggested in 1971, "as a legitimizing mechanism for enacting or originating policy."[3] I will find this out when the report of the Royal Commission is released.

NOTES

1   Meekosha, Helen, "Research and the State: Dilemmas of Feminist Practice." *Australian Journal of Social Issues* 24 (1989): 250.

2   Meekosha, p. 258.

3   Horowitz, Irving L., *The Use and Abuse of Social Science: Behavioral Science and National Policy Making.* New Brunswick, New Jersey: Transaction Books, 1971, p.4.

ANONYMOUS 5

WHY I WON'T WRITE ABOUT MY EXPERIENCES WORKING WITH THE ROYAL COMMISSION ON NEW REPRODUCTIVE TECHNOLOGIES — OR: SILENCED SURVIVORS

There are many of us, I think, who would like to speak candidly about our experiences working for the Royal Commission on New Reproductive Technologies (RCNRT), but we don't. What power is held over us, even now, when we have long ago shredded the last "confidential" file, deleted a final incriminating e-mail or hidden in our briefcase a damning memo or secret document? Even among ourselves we are cautious, for fear that a mole has infiltrated our secret club of the silenced survivors. Why after all this time do we continue to censor ourselves?

A partial answer to this question is rooted in the reign of terror which governed the workplace, arousing paranoia and distrust in many of us and eroding our sense of solidarity and commitment. As some of us were to be told at a Commission wide staff meeting, ours was a Darwinian Commission. "If you can't cut it then you're out, it's very Darwinian you know!" What this meant in practice however, had nothing to do with "cutting it" professionally or intellectually. Survival was not achieved by the fittest — many of those were "let go." Those of us who did "cut it" for a while at least, survived because we played it safe on the outside, all the while raging inside. We managed to retain our jobs, for a while, at the expense of our emotional and psychological well-being. We also thought it important to have representation on the inside, so that accounts like these could be told, hopefully in the future, with more detail. We were, by then, beyond the point of hoping that our presence could make a difference with regard to the "work" that was being produced by the Commission — ours was to be a different sort of legacy.

Many of us who joined the Commission as analysts and researchers soon after its inception came with a particular expertise and staunch commitment to the interdisciplinary investigation of the multitude of issues raised by the mandate of the RCNRT. We were sociologists, lawyers, historians, nurses, epidemiologists, politcal scientists, public health specialists, economists and, in a few cases, civil servants. Almost all of us were women. For most of us, this was more than a job. It was to have been an extraordinary opportunity to generate an original body of research about a subject matter with enormous ethical, social, personal and political implications. We were dedicated to fashioning social policy which would be responsive to the magnitude and complexity of the issues. This, however, meant that not only were the medical and "scientific" issues to be canvassed and reckoned with, but that a sophisticated investigation of the myriad of social, legal and ethical issues also needed to be undertaken. It meant that medical and scientific issues could be analyzed in a different way — there is no consensus even in these communities about them. In addition, because of the gender dimension to the various forms of reproductive technologies we were of the view (as, apparently, was the Federal government which appointed the Commission and instructed it to pay particular attention to issues as they affected women) that the implications of various practices and techniques for women should also be investigated. And, because women (and men) are not a monolithic category but flesh and blood individuals variously situated, we were also committed to an investigation of social diversity. What were the differential impacts of the various technologies on various racial and ethnic groups, on gays and lesbians, for those differently positioned on the socio-economic scale, for those living in rural communities and for the disabled? This was a challenging research agenda requiring a novel interdisciplinary plan of action.

Sadly however, the powers that be had a different agenda. From the outset, the conventional medical model of research prevailed, augmented with a rigid hierarchical bureaucratic structure. Frankenstein meets Kafka. Discrete medical and scientific categories structured the Research Working Groups: Infertility; Assisted Reproduction; Genetic Testing and Screening; and Embryo and Fetal Tissue Research. The technologies drove the research categories and any other classification of research subject was rejected. No wonder the last year of the Commission has been spent "filling gaps." Moreover, the privileged methodology was that of the scientific model. Projects which could not yield "hard" data were not conducted or regarded as highly suspect. The scientific paradigm was the norm to which everything else was to aspire. Facts could only be objectively produced through this method. But human interaction and social data are more complicated than this and not so easily reduced to quantifiable or observable data.

The research and analysis branches of the Commission were physically and bureaucratically separated. Moreover, in predictable bureaucratic fashion the two sections worked in competition rather than in cooperation with each other. This dichotomy between research and analysis was a symbolic representation of the way in which research and policy making were to be carried on by the Commission. The fact/value distinction was built into the very institutional structure of the Commission. Somehow, it was assumed that Research could produce "the facts" — objective, neutral and truthful — and the Analysis would and could distill meaning from them in an "ice cold" fashion, of course. Another favoured project of the Analysis section was to "analyze" the reports and recommendations of various international and national commissions and committees which had already investigated issues similar to those being examined by the RCNRT. This was a sensible undertaking, however such analyses were to be nothing more than a summary of the conclusions of each report. No true analyses were to take place.

For all the pretense about generating an accurate factual basis upon which to base policy proposals and recommendations, perhaps the most disturbing occurrence to take place at the Commission was an oft stated phrase: "the data could be massaged." As I write this now, not long before the long anticipated

Final Report is to be delivered, I wonder which will have been more massaged: the data or the oh so fragile egos of certain members of the Commission and their dutiful staff. It has been a terrible disappointment.

ANONYMOUS 6

The disappointment after working at the Royal Commission on New Reproductive Technologies is a difficult emotion to explain. Perhaps I could just say that now, some time later, I still have nightmares about my experiences at the Commission.

What a shame that a Commission that had so much promise for quality debate and productive discussion turned into such a limited and paranoid environment. I took the job, like most of us, due to the fascinating subject matter. The issues, whether new reproductive technologies should be covered under medicare, and the myriad of social, legal, economic, political, feminist, medical and scientific issues that I thought were going to be discussed at the Commission, was a definite draw to the job.

It is difficult to unravel exactly what went wrong. What I had thought would be a stimulating, exciting work environment turned out to be an apathetic, uninterested and generally unhappy group of people. When attempts were made to organize meetings or meet with people to discuss ideas, one always had to be careful that one was not talking to the "wrong" person, for some people just could not be trusted. Who exactly those people were always hung heavy on one's mind. Having come from a background where discussion and deep analysis is encouraged, I had to "learn" to hold my tongue and not always give my honest opinion as it might have been seen as threatening.

Nothing was predictable at the Commission. I believe that this was really what made it into a reign of terror. People who never appeared to have problems were fired at the last moment, and no one ever heard of them again. Rumours were spread about someone's behaviour or ideas that were "problematic." I myself, found out that my e-mails had been broken into and a friend of mine became so fearful that she suspected that her home telephone was being tapped.

I was asked recently whether I believe that this scandal took place as a result of the theme — new reproductive technologies. On reflection I think that this is only partially true. Any subject requiring a Royal Commission is bound to be controversial, for that is why the in-depth reflection of a commission is required. However, I believe that two factors stand out. The staff at the Directorial and Deputy Directorial levels were indifferent and smug about the issue (and about people in general), and difference of opinion on any subject was neither encouraged nor tolerated. This is not normal. And secondly, there is big money at stake in the future of new reproductive technologies. Pharmaceutical companies (and associates) and private practitioners were closely linked to some of the work executed at the Royal Commission so the non-medical points of view were not highly respected (to say the least).

What is truly sad about the Royal Commission on New Reproductive Technologies, however, is not so much that people like myself suffered, and that we are still licking our wounds, but more importantly, that the issue of new reproductive technologies has still not been given a fair hearing. And furthermore, the issue of women's reproductive health is once again being managed by forces too powerful to control.

14

THE PUBLIC HEARINGS OF THE ROYAL COMMISSION ON NEW REPRODUCTIVE TECHNOLOGIES: AN EVALUATION

Christine Massey

The Royal Commission on New Reproductive Technologies was called upon to fulfil two of the most common tasks for royal commissions — first, to offer an opportunity for public involvement in the policy process and second, to provide an assessment of scientific and technological developments.[1] The Commission offered its "total society" approach to public participation to deal with the complexities of a technologically-informed and scientifically intricate debate. How effective was the Commission in attracting and involving the public in a process that allowed the public's values and opinions to reflect upon the science and new technologies in question?

WHAT IS PUBLIC PARTICIPATION?

Sherry Arnstein probably distilled the goal of public participation to its most fundamental element when she wrote, "citizen participation is... citizen power."[2] Although public participation is considered central to our system of democracy, most of our experiences with public involvement in policy-making fall short of actual power sharing; they are truly just "exercises" — all process and no substance.

Decisions involving science and technology pose a special challenge for public involvement efforts because the public has never been considered a legitimate partner and contributor to science and technology policies.[3] The assumed authority and objectivity of scientists and experts is such that science can replace democratic decision making; decisions can be supported by scientific studies alone. Special interest groups, defending social and human values, are perceived as less "objective" and less able to contribute to a discussion over scientific and technological risks.[4] This monopoly of knowledge and status effectively obscures issues of power; the exclusion of the public is given a rational basis.

PUBLIC PARTICIPATION IN ROYAL COMMISSIONS

Royal commissions are often created and defended on the grounds that they provide an open and impartial way to assess policy options.[5] The Inquiries Act, under which most royal commissions are created, offers no standards for the holding of public hearings beyond authorizing the commission to subpoena witnesses. A publication widely regarded as the "Bible" of commission management[6] devotes a total of two pages to the conduct of hearings and is primarily concerned with proper procedures, not effective participation.[7] In large part, the format, structure, content and timing of public participation is left up to the discretion of the inquiry commissioners.[8] As a result, commissioners have a great deal of freedom in structuring public participation to suit whatever goals they choose.

Unfortunately, royal commissions seem to be bound (whether by law or tradition is unclear) to the public hearing as a means of involving the public. Although toll-free telephone lines, written submissions or letters have also been used, the hearing remains the most consistent and preferred method. Yet, public hearings, as a technique of public participation, have some serious weaknesses. Some of the most common drawbacks are: procedural rules which make it difficult to initiate two-way communication; intervenors who are not representative of the total population; and the lack of impact on the final decision.[9] Abuses to which the public hearing lends itself are: a habit of inadequate notification; the selective or elite involvement in the hearings; and an overemphasis on providing information rather than receiving it.[10]

While the above describes the historical trend with respect to public hearings, there have been some more successful uses of the technique. The Mackenzie Valley Pipeline Inquiry, chaired by then B.C. Supreme Court Justice

Thomas Berger in the mid-70s, has achieved international attention and acclaim for its efforts at integrating in an evenhanded way, technical, political and social testimony, primarily through the use of innovative, unconventional and informal community hearings.[11] The testimony gathered from the community hearings regarding native culture, traditions and knowledge of the area was allowed as evidence on par with the technical submissions from the pipeline company.[12]

The work of the Berger Commission points to the significant potential that royal commissions have to give voice to radical marginal groups who would otherwise have no standing in the course of the normal political process.[13] Unfortunately, the Berger Commission seems to be the exception that proves the rule; in practice, this potential is rarely fully realized.

More commonly, royal commissions give voice and legitimacy to those groups in our society who already have it. While all intervenors may officially be equals in the hearings process, those with a financial and/or legal interest in the issue tend to be given greater status. Advocacy groups, especially those with more diffuse memberships, suffer most. Their claims, based on far-ranging, less defined and fundamental principles, are viewed as less legitimate than claims made on the basis of specific rights well established in our legal system (for example, property rights).[14] This devaluation of "non-experts" is only further compounded when the issue in question is also a scientific one.

The fact that royal commissions operate in ways that favour established patterns of decision-making should come as no surprise to us if we consider that these are bodies appointed by governments in power. Inquiries must operate within a web of political institutions and agencies, departments and cabinets, many of which have more decision-making power than the inquiry itself.[15] As a result, inquiries act best as mirrors to what is going on outside them.[16] The tendency is for these pressures to prevail and for old patterns to be perpetuated. As Richard Simeon writes of royal commissions, "By their very nature, they can be no more than meliorative and reformist, rather than revolutionary."[17]

As a final point, one of the reasons that royal commissions have had such an uneven history is due to the central role of the commissioners or commission chair in determining the purpose and form of a commission's work. The very issues which are at the root of many inquiry participants' complaints — the procedures to be used, the inquiry priorities, and what questions are up for discussion — are those which are controlled by the commissioners.[18] Although the precise definition of the problem or crisis to be examined is often the most crucial decision of a public inquiry, it is not regularly an open part of the commission work and not subject to public input and control. This decision has enormous implications for the kind of debate that will ensue, the type of research that will be sought out and the kind of proposals that will be given serious consideration as final recommendations.[19] Any and all the improvements in the process of public participation will be countered by this basic concentration of decision-making power in a single person or a few people.

PUBLIC PARTICIPATION IN THE ROYAL COMMISSION ON NEW REPRODUCTIVE TECHNOLOGIES[20]

The Royal Commission on New Reproductive Technologies was called upon to evaluate and assess not only future advances in new reproductive technologies (NRTs) but ones that had already been made widely available to the public. In Canada, the first clinic for sex preselection opened in Toronto in 1987; the Royal Commission on New Reproductive Technologies was announced in 1989. While the scientific and technological work had gone ahead, the Commission was expected to follow with an ethical evaluation for policy purposes. Already the Commission was faced with a situation with significant interests at stake which could seriously circumscribe the kind of policy options available. The economic and scientific investment in these technologies is such that any opposition on the part of public groups would require the development of a substantial "critical mass" of public opinion and action.

Although precise global figures of the economic interests in NRTs are notoriously difficult to obtain, some partial figures can give us a good idea. If we take in vitro fertilization (IVF) as an example, the cost of drugs for one cycle of IVF (and the vast majority of women need more than one cycle) is about US$ 1600. Ares-Serono, one of the leading firms in the area of fertility drugs used for

IVF, recorded revenues of $260 million internationally in 1991 from the sale of these drugs. These sales, however, are just the tip of the iceberg if one considers IVF specialist Dr. Bernard Lunenfeld's estimate of the potential market in the industrialized world for fertility drugs: 10 million women, joined every year thereafter by an additional 700,000.[21]

In planning for public participation, the Commission was presumably faced with a series of choices in structuring its public participation process. According to its public announcements, the Commission fully intended to involve the public in its investigation:

> *The Commission...has set up an extensive Public Consultations Program to give Canadians from all walks of life and from all regions of the country the opportunity to contribute to the work, as it studies the origins, effects and impacts of the technologies.*[22]

In seeking public opinion and input on the NRTs, the Royal Commission did not have an immediately obvious public constituency to call upon. There were no "NRT" advocacy groups in the manner that Energy Probe would be an advocacy group for nuclear power issues. The intimate nature of the topic was such that individuals with personal experience of infertility and treatment would not be likely to discuss these issues in a public forum (although several people, to their credit, did). As for the women's movement, while many of Canada's women's groups had begun to do some work on the issue, NRTs were still a new and emerging issue that suffered from a significant lack of information. Furthermore, NRTs could be only one focus of the ever expanding agenda of "women's issues" in which these chronically underfunded groups are involved.

Women's groups were not the only organizations to undertake work on NRTs on behalf of their group's interest. For example, visible minority groups expanded their agendas to include the political ramifications of the development of NRTs. However, these advocacy groups, including women's groups, are frequently volunteer organizations with few resources. Some found it difficult to develop enough expertise in a new area to present their concerns to an official body, especially in the short time allotted. (Public hearings were announced May of 1990. Although the initial deadline for requests to appear was the end of July 1990, this date had to be extended due to protests.) Diverting valuable staff, volunteers and resources to an entirely new and complicated area was a tough decision for some groups and often depended on the dedication of effort by a single individual.

The only evident and ready constituencies that the Commission was assured of were the medical and research communities, the pharmaceutical industry and the legal profession. IVF clinics, their doctors, researchers in hospitals, universities and private practice represented the most experienced people in the subject area and with their greater access to funds, could more easily prepare official submissions. These groups were also represented by their well funded national professional associations, among them, the Society of Obstetricians and Gynaecologists of Canada, the Royal College of Physicians and Surgeons of Canada and the Canadian Medical Association. These intervenors carried with them the traditional authority of science as well as the weight of their financial interests in the technologies (usually left unsaid) which, as discussed above, are supported and granted greater legitimacy in an inquiry setting than are advocacy groups with their more qualitative concerns.

While many doctors, clinicians and researchers did present at the hearings, it is equally evident that some prominent stakeholders chose not to participate, among them the Pharmaceutical Manufacturer's Association and the individual pharmaceutical firms. (Organon Canada submitted only a written brief.) The choice of these firms not to appear at the hearings is curious given their significant investment in the drugs used in many of the NRTs. This decision suggests that either they considered the hearings an inappropriate forum to promote their views or that they were aware of better ways of making their interests known to the Commission. Perhaps both.

Certainly, the absence of industry representatives from the hearings could not be ignored by the Commission, and in fact, private consultations with these parties were initiated after the public hearings were over.[23] The groundwork for these consultations was, however, contracted to a public relations firm, Burson-Marsteller, a company which counts among its clients several pharmaceutical firms.[24] Apart from the conflict of interest involved in the choice of this firm, the use of public relations experts points to an approach to consultation that favours image over substance and placation over debate.

Without an obvious public constituency, the Commission could have opted for a series of preliminary hearings in the manner of the Berger Commission. Preliminary hearings provide a forum for the exploration of the needs of possible participants as well as for a negotiation over the priorities for the public debate to follow in the hearings stage. Groups can apply for intervenor funding. The opportunity to meet can also point to how different groups can benefit by pooling resources and working together. Unfortunately, this option was not chosen and the information, funding and time needs of many groups went unexpressed.

As it was, the mobilization of all of these groups, while normally the task of the Royal Commission, was partly due to the work of other organizations. The Coalition for a Royal Commission on New Reproductive Technologies made considerable efforts to encourage various organizations to get involved. The New Democrat Member of Parliament, Dawn Black, sent a message to over 4000 individual women and women's groups outlining the steps to take to become involved. And finally, many groups made use of the then recently published Canadian Research Institute for the Advancement of Women's guide to the NRTs.

Even without the benefit of preliminary hearings, in approaching a subject like the reproductive technologies, the Commission must have been aware of the barriers to effective public understanding posed by the scientific language and technical details. Advocacy groups new to the topic found it a challenge to decipher the "scientific jargon" and to then become familiar enough with it to make an official presentation to a government body.

One participant prepared a brief despite what she found to be the overwhelming amount of scientific data to learn and the intimidating thought of presenting herself to a royal commission. Her presentation reflected the thoughts, no doubt, of many Canadians — it ran through a variety of techniques, highlighting the many questions and ethical concerns raised by the procedures.

To her dismay, the first reaction to her brief from a commissioner was the rather dismissive question, "So you aren't making any recommendations are you?"

This incident is not meant to be unfair to commissioners, who, no doubt, found it a challenge to hear, for example, a technical submission from an IVF clinic doctor immediately followed by the very personal and perhaps less focused thoughts of a woman experiencing fertility problems. In this, the Commission could have learned from the Berger experience where separate hearings were held for technical submissions and for communities, public groups and interested individuals. Each type of hearing allows for a discussion of both social issues and technological issues (which are inseparable) but in the language and format in which each group is most comfortable.

Another way of encouraging public debate on a new and scientific issue is to conduct a public education campaign directed towards the general public and aimed at increasing awareness of the issues and problems. No such significant public education campaign was undertaken by the Royal Commission beyond the distribution of information kits to certain groups and to those who requested them.

These kits included a pamphlet published to encourage participation as well as to familiarize the public with the issues that the Commission expected to address.[25] The pamphlet is presented as a primer for a newcomer to the subject of NRTs. A question and answer format is used, where an imaginary reader's questions are presumed, provided and then answered — a model, perhaps, for the entire public consultation process. The pamphlet provides no explanation of the procedures in question, no statistics (i.e., costs, success rates, prevalence) and indicates no other sources for more information on different subjects. The summary attempts to provide balance by offering various interpretations of the technologies, including the critiques of the technologies that led to the initial demands for a Royal Commission. However, without the necessary context or information, questions such as: "to what extent do the various technologies create conditions which do or could exploit women,"[26] appear curiously unfounded and isolated.

The Royal Commission information kit seems especially lacking when it is compared to a similar kit produced at the same time by the Canadian Research

Institute for the Advancement of Women.[27] This kit consisted of a series of separate information sheets that explained the technologies and processes involved in NRTs and the debate that had arisen around each of them. It also provided advice on seeking more information and resources on various topics, on facilitating discussions and on preparing a brief for the Royal Commission. Also included was a glossary of scientific terms related to NRTs. For those new to the issue of NRTs, the kit truly provided the tools that could lead to a successful intervention in the Commission's work.

Instead of a public information campaign to develop awareness and knowledge for the most effective public participation, the Commission ordered public opinion polls. A national poll was conducted to determine the attitudes of Canadians toward NRTs. Another survey was done of Canadian ethnocultural communities.[28] Unfortunately, a poll which questions people on complex scientific and ethical issues about which they know little, is no substitute for participation. Polling is a passive form of political participation, where the kind of questions deemed important, their context and the range of possible alternatives are determined by the poll designers, according to their goals.[29] This is quite different from engaging in a shared process of decision-making with citizens, where citizens are genuine partners in determining their public policies.

The first national poll conducted by the Commission was assessed by one of the fired Commissioners who opposed it on the grounds that its method was unsound and that the questions tended towards misinformation (for example, by suggesting that NRTs were successful treatments for infertility).[30] Nonetheless, the Royal Commission included those survey respondents in calculations of their rate of public participation:

> More than 40,000 Canadians from across the country participated in clinical studies and national surveys, attended Public Hearings and Private Sessions, sent letters of opinion or written submissions, or left their thoughts on our toll-free telephone lines.[31]

This same figure appeared in another, later edition of *Update* without the corresponding explanation.[32] To include subjects of clinical studies and survey respondents in figures of public participation suggests a vision of citizen involvement that is limited at best, passive and easily manipulated at worst.

Another variation on the public education campaign is for a commission to provide an on-going summary of its hearings to the interested community and for the benefit of future participants. For example, the Berger Commission arranged with the Northern CBC radio service to have its hearings summarized daily. This Commission instead chose to depend on the mass media to communicate to the public the issues emerging during the hearings. Unfortunately, the combination of deadlines, a generalist education and scarce resources make it difficult for the average reporter to be able to represent a complex scientific issue to its fullest. Usually only one or two opposing views around a particular issue are discussed and these are made to fit into reliable story "pegs." One of these story pegs is conflict and the following examples point to the inadequacy of relying solely upon the mass media to foster sober debate.

The press coverage of the hearings in Toronto during October of 1990 characterized the debate as the "feminists" vs. the "infertile." Feminists, primarily represented by the National Action Committee on the Status of Women (NAC), were portrayed as denying "choice" to infertile women who, in turn, were desperate to try anything to conceive.[33] The emphasis on the conflict was such that the NAC felt compelled to reply in letters to the editor, and another smaller group of women who presented at the last set of hearings in Vancouver, also felt compelled to structure their brief as a correction of the press coverage.[34]

The media coverage of the Vancouver hearings was focused on the presentation of Dr. Stephens, who had quite publicly directed his sex-preselection clinic to South Asian women. Coverage represented the story as a conflict between Dr. Stephens and South Asian women picketing outside. While this conflict did exist, many other issues were discussed at these hearings, none of which received attention.[35]

The public hearings of the Royal Commission were organized as a forum where commissioners would make themselves available to hear the submissions of any who wished to appear. This format attempts to be less like a court room than other kinds of inquiry hearings; no cross-examination of witnesses is allowed although questions of clarification may be posed by the commissioners or their staff. The process is designed as a one-way flow of information from intervenors to commissioners; it is not a forum for public debate.

Unfortunately, it also appears as if the Commission did not place much faith in the public hearing even as a one-way mode of communication. Commissioners participated in "media and public relations" seminars designed to prepare them for the public hearings. Commissioners were taught how to yawn without appearing to and how to give the impression of listening when tired.[36]

Even the most sincere efforts of a commissioner to give intervenors his or her full attention cannot overcome the major disadvantage to this type of hearing — the lack of a single public forum for the pulling together of public views for debate. Intervenors cannot address the arguments made by others unless they have attended all the hearings. Most of the real work is done by inquiry staff after the submissions have been presented and the analysis is done.[37]

The hearings were held in hotel ballrooms in major urban centres across the country, a traditional arena for royal commission hearings. The lay-out of the rooms was similarly quite formal. The Commissioners sat at a large head table, separated by a large distance from a smaller table where the intervenors sat. This kind of room lay-out communicates a clear message to intervenors regarding the distribution of power between commissioners and intervenors.

It should be noted that the format and structure of the public hearings constituted one of the subjects of contention in the lawsuit laid against Patricia Baird and the Government by the four Commissioners, Bruce Hatfield, Martin Hébert, Maureen McTeer and Louise Vandelac. They claimed that the public hearings process, designed without their input, prevented them,

> ...from truly pursuing the important matters raised by intervening individuals and groups, forcing them instead to resort to a limited and superficial discussion with intervenors, focusing on the form rather than the substance of the process.[38]

The hearings were held only in major urban centres without any provisions for travel allowances or child care (a surprising omission considering the topic under discussion), a decision which no doubt excluded many rural women's groups as well as aboriginal groups. Of course, it is difficult to guess at what might have been had resources been available, but of the 250 organizations who appeared before the Commission, only two represented aboriginal women.[39] Perhaps in an effort to make up for the inadequacies of the initial effort, the Commission held a roundtable discussion with aboriginal women in the North.[40] Unfortunately, this consultation would not address the views and needs of aboriginal women on reserves across the country, whose special circumstances and health concerns would no doubt affect infertility rates and questions of access.

The Commission did not fail to recognize the lack of participation from many types of groups in its public hearings. An internal Commission memo points to a lack of input from, "industry, the francophone community, various ethnocultural communities, youth, religious groups and aboriginals."[41] According to the memo's author, the lack of input from these groups stemmed not from an inadequate information campaign or the lack of an accessible process but, "because they had nothing to say on our mandate or because they did not understand the issues or our process."[42]

At this point, it should be noted that, notwithstanding the history of government consultation exercises and the extra demand on resources that participation entailed, a number of groups, particularly voluntary ones, took the time and effort to appear with well-reasoned critiques and proposals. This fact can serve as testimony to the significance placed on NRTs by many in Canada as well as the continued faith in democratic principles. Many of these participants felt quite simply compelled by the magnitude of the issue to make some sort of representation to the Commission.

In all, the public hearings, although spread over three months, took 28 days. As a proportion of the Commission's total mandate (October 1989-July 1993) this process was quite brief. At the least, it offers a gauge as to how much importance the Commission accorded public input.

The Commission engaged in other techniques of seeking public information, among them a toll-free telephone line, written submissions and letters and the more innovative private sessions for those with intimate experiences with the technologies.[43] Unfortunately, these techniques suffer from the same failing as the public hearings in that none of them provides for a collection and debate of public views in a single (or series of) discussions. These strategies were all dependent on the initiative of citizens to contact the Commission and in this respect, must be evaluated in light of the lack of public awareness and an education campaign.

Furthermore, there is little indication as to how this information will be incorporated into the final report. Liora Salter, an observer of the drafting of inquiry reports, relates how this process, conducted in private, resembles more a negotiation than an assessment. While the government is often present at the table "in spirit" as commissioners attempt to gauge what will be accepted and ignored in the form of recommendations, there is no equal presence for the various views presented by different public groups during the hearings. This loss of public accountability at this stage often leads to the inappropriate use of comments from public submissions and research, out of context, to support the various commission recommendations.[44]

Public hearings are one way of ensuring accountability for a royal commission. Unfortunately, for a Commission explicitly directed to consider women's health and well-being, participants from small, local women's groups felt excluded. They were dismayed over what seemed to be an inappropriately formal and expensive hearings process, and a general lack of meaningful consultation that left them without any input into guiding the priorities of the Commission. Without this kind of necessary transparency, the Royal Commission on New Reproductive Technologies proceeded in a highly traditional and limited manner. The experts in this process were the doctors, scientists and lawyers, not the grassroots organizations who deal with and represent women on a day-to-day basis.

CONCLUSION

When considering royal commissions as a site for achieving significant progress in the realm of public participation, one can point to certain exceptional efforts — the Berger Commission or the Bird Commission on the Status of Women. On the whole, however, the royal commission cannot be depended on as a progressive body for public involvement. Royal commissions, as state-created institutions, headed by privileged members of society (lawyers and academics make up a substantial proportion of all royal commission memberships) are unlikely to be revolutionary instruments of citizen control. Rather, they are exercises in "mandated participation"[45] — opportunities for participation predetermined by the state and made available under state control. As such, any efforts at participation will be limited because the control of the process lies entirely with the government and resides in the commission chair.

The Royal Commission on New Reproductive Technologies had the same potential as all commissions to include a wide variety of voices in its deliberations. By not taking action to address the difficulties of public involvement in science policy, the Commission's hearings fell short of their potential. The Commission did not attend to the particular needs of public groups who wanted to be a part of the process or seek innovative and effective methods of participation. The result was to privilege the scientific and legal experts and to miss an opportunity to engage in fruitful public discussion around a complex scientific issue.

NOTES

1   Liora Salter and Debra Slaco. *Public Inquiries in Canada*, Ottawa: Supply and Services, 1981 p.21-2

2   Sherry Arnstein. "A Ladder of Public Participation" *Journal of the American Institute of Planners* vol.35 no.4 July 1968 p.216

3   Organisation for Economic Co-operation and Development (OECD). *Technology on Trial: Public Participation in Decision-Making Related to Science and Technology.* Paris: OECD, 1979 p.7

4   For a critique of the ideal of the scientific method and its use in developing and maintaining the authority of science see, for example: Barry Barnes and David Edge (eds) *Science in Context* Cambridge: The MIT Press, 1982; Margaret Benston "Feminism and the Critique of the Scientific Method" in *Feminism: From Pressure to Politics* A.R. Miles and G.Finn (eds) Montreal: Black Rose Books, 1989; R.C. Lewontin. *Biology as Ideology.* Concord, Ontario: Anansi, 1991; Michael Mulkay *Science and the Sociology of Knowledge.* Boston: George Allen & Unwin, 1979.

5   Sylvia Bashevkin. "Does public opinion matter? The adoption of federal royal commission and task force recommendations on the national question, 1951-1987." *Canadian Public Administration.* vol.31 no.1 Fall 1988 p.391

6   A. Wayne MacKay. "Mandates, Legal Foundations, Power and Conduct of Commissions of Inquiry" *Commissions of Inquiry* A. Paul Pross, Innis Christie, John A. Yogis (eds.) Toronto: Carswell, 1990 p.35

7   Harry A. Wilson. *Commissions of Inquiry: A Handbook of Operations.* Ottawa: Privy Council Office, 1983 p.31-2

8   Russell J. Anthony and Alastair R. Lucas. *A Handbook on the Conduct of Public Inquiries in Canada.* Toronto: Butterworths, 1985 p.52

9   Barry Checkoway. "The Politics of Public Hearings." *The Journal of Applied Behavioral Science*. vol.14 no.4 1981 p.566-581.

10 Gregory A. Daneke "Introduction" *Public Involvement and Social Impact Assessment* Gregory A. Daneke, Margot W. Garcia and Jerome Delli Priscoli (eds) Boulder, CO: Westview Press, 1983 p.17

11 OECD, 1979 p.68-75

12 *Ibid*. p.69-71

13 Liora Salter "The Two Contradictions in Public Inquiries" *Commissions of Inquiry*. A.Paul Pross, Innis Christie and John A. Yogis (eds.) Toronto: Carswell, 1990 p.175-5

14 *Ibid*. p.187-192

15 *Ibid*. p.221

16 Salter and Slaco 1981 p.15

17 Richard Simeon. "Inside the MacDonald Commission" *Studies in Political Economy*. vol.22 1987 p.169

18 John J. Rodger. "Natural justice and the big public inquiry: a sociological perspective" *Sociological Review*. vol.33 no.3 August 1985 p.411

19 Salter 1990 p.182

20 Many of the observations in this section come from personal interviews with intervenors in the public hearings process.

21 Ares-Serono profits, *New York Times* 19 April 1992, sec.F; Varda Burstyn, "Breeding Discontent," *Saturday Night*, June 1993, p.65.

22 Royal Commission on New Reproductive Technologies "Royal Commission takes 'total society' approach to new reproductive technologies." press release, 1990.

23 Royal Commission on New Reproductive Technologies *Update* Aug. 1992 p.10

24 Contract, dated October 1, 1991 between the Royal Commission on New Reproductive Technologies and Burson-Marsteller, RCNRT document #91-C-060; Varda Burstyn, cited in "Panel too close to pharmaceutical firms, groups says," Vancouver *Sun*. February 4, 1992.

25 Royal Commission on New Reproductive Technologies. A Guide to Public Participation in the Work of the Royal Commission on New Reproductive Technologies. January 1991.

26 *Ibid*. p.10

27 Canadian Research Institute for the Advancement of Women, "Our Bodies, Our Babies? Women Look at New Reproductive Technologies." Ottawa: CRIAW, November 1989.

28 Royal Commission on New Reproductive Technologies. *Update* August 1992 p.9

29 Benjamin Ginsberg, *The Captive Public*. New York: Basic Books, 1989. pp.59-85.

30 This assessment can be consulted as part of the Statement of Claim (document #T303591) laid in Federal Court, Trial Division, Ottawa, December 6, 1991 by Bruce Hatfield, Martin Hébert, Maureen McTeer, and Louise Vandelac vs. the Queen, the Attorney of Canada and Patricia Baird. Schedule 20.

31 Royal Commission on New Reproductive Technologies *Update* August 1992 p.1

32 Royal Commission on New Reproductive Technologies. *Update*. November 1992

33 See for example: Toronto *Star* October 29, 1990 p.A2 and October 30 1990 p.A3. *Globe and Mail* October 29 1990 p.A5 and October 30 1990 p.A4. Also Montreal *Gazette* Nov. 22 1990 p.A6. Toronto *Star* Nov.20 1990 p.A11, *Globe and Mail* Nov.21 1990 p.A10 and Nov. 23 1990 p.A2.

34 NAC's response: Globe and Mail Nov.24 1990 p.D7. Brief presented to the Royal Commission on New Reproductive Technologies by the Vancouver Women's Reproductive Technologies Coalition.

35 See for example, Vancouver *Sun* Nov.27 1990 p.A1, Ottawa *Citizen* Nov.27 1990 p. A3, Toronto *Star* Nov.27 1990 p.A10. *Globe and Mail* Nov.15 1990 p.A8

36 Louise Vandelac. Presentation to the National Association of Women and the Law Tenth Biennial Conference. Vancouver, February 20, 1993.

37 Anthony and Lucas 1985 p.67

38 Statement of Claim (document #T303591) laid in Federal Court, Trial Division, Ottawa, December 6, 1991 by Bruce Hatfield, Martin Hébert, Maureen McTeer and Louise Vandelac vs. the Queen, the Attorney of Canada and Patricia Baird. Article 51.

39 Indian and Inuit Nurses of Canada, Yukon Indian Women's Association.

40 Royal Commission on New Reproductive Technologies, *Update* August 1992 p.11

41 Memorandum to Commissioners, Re: Organization Consultations August 20, 1991. Can be consulted as part of the Federal Court Statement of Claim, Schedule 20.

42 *Ibid*

43 Royal Commission on New Reproductive Technologies *Update*, August 1992 p.8-11

44 Salter 1990 p.183

45 I am indebted to Dr. Catherine Murray, Department of Communication, Simon Fraser University, for this term as well as many other insights.

15

THE BAIRD COMMISSION: FROM 'ACCESS' TO 'REPRODUCTIVE TECHNOLOGIES' TO THE 'EXCESSES' OF PRACTITIONERS OR THE ART OF DIVERSION AND RELENTLESS PURSUIT...

Louise Vandelac

"In the past 'power' meant land — control over what grew on it and what was extracted from it. Then 'power' came to mean manufacturing — traditional industries. Today, 'power' is life... and 'life' is becoming the private grounds of transnationals and risk capital investors."[1]

At the dawn of the 21st century, the reproductive technologies have the power not only to transform human conception now and in the future, but to alter the very nature of medicine. This human "branch" of the new "industry of life" has, in fact, the power to transform our very concept of humanity. It is in the context of these transformations and the redefinition of power to which they lead that the extraordinary secrecy and the unbelievable authoritarianism of the Baird Commission and its use of the media can best be understood.

INTRODUCTION

April 1993. The media, responding to Dr. Patricia Baird's press conference on "fertility programs" in Canada, condemn the Chair of the Royal Commission on New Reproductive Technologies for her lack of judgment. The word "irresponsible" is used by several people to describe the Commission's silence for almost one year about the risk of AIDS transmission from the use of sperm from non-tested donors for artificial insemination, and its refusal to reveal the names of the doctors and clinics involved. Commentators considered it cynical, to say the least, that after four years of work costing more than $25 million, Dr. Baird should content herself with merely urging women to be careful and to question their doctors.

The media outburst lasted about a week. The press gave both Baird and the Commission a rough ride and they temporarily lost a little more credibility. But soon everything seemed to be back to normal — notwithstanding a few more waves in July when it was announced, for the third time, that the final report of the Commission would again be postponed.[2]

This most recent management of blunders and delays by the Commission is evidence of what we can expect when the final report is released: polished image creation by the Commission as it shifts the focus from access to the New Reproductive Technologies (NRTs) to a new issue, control of excesses, followed by a positive reception from the media and general approval of its recommendations. At most, there may be some criticism of the Commission in the media, but, if the past is a guide, thoughtful analyses of the issues will be absent.

POLITICS, SCIENCE, GENETICS AND MANIPULATION

Is it paradoxical to predict the report's "success?" Is it paradoxical to maintain, months before its release as this is being written, that the report will seduce the press to the point where it will forego any critical analysis, any investigative work?[3]

As an ex-commissioner on that Kafkaesque Commission, I saw up close how words could be twisted and drained of meaning. This is why I believe that the analytical framework and the terms in which the debate on reproductive technologies have been and will be set down by the Commission are booby-trapped, clouding, when not blocking, our thinking on these matters. Remember that the dominant discourse about NRTs comes from authorities who, despite their multidisciplinary backgrounds,[4] are based in the world of biomedicine. Claiming that these technologies are medical, and framing them as ways to deal with problems (re)classified as medical, these authorities have, for the most part, supported the transformation of childbearing, while the few more critical voices have gone unheeded.[5]

In Canada, representatives of the biomedical profession have tried to frame the discourse with their presentations to the media and to the Commission. Already, the recommendations of the Society of Obstetricians and Gynecologists of Canada (SOGC) which, as we shall see, may at times have more the appearance than the reality of an ethical analysis, clearly open the way to commercial trade in gametes, embryos and childbearing; to the privatization of "artificial reproduction services"; and to the public and private funding of research on gametes and embryos. As well, Dr. Baird, a pediatrician and geneticist herself inspired by these same approaches, has dominated the media and political discussion for years. While she has not seemed able to make the time during her four years at the Commission to inform the public appropriately about either the nature or current status of the technologies and practices,[6] or to initiate a genuine public debate on the genesis and the social effects of these technologies, she seems nonetheless to have succeeded in imposing an analytical framework that takes most of the practices for granted — without, of course, examining their validity or significance. The tasks remaining for her, therefore, are only to legitimize the technologies or encourage their diffusion, insuring only that the most marginal are brushed aside while the remainder — or at least their excesses — are managed.

This approach is a hoax, capitalizing on the general esteem given to medicine. It reduces the radical transformation of childbearing and the new production of "living laboratories"[7] to questions of efficiency and consumption.

Further, the kind of individualist and consumerist perspective that dominates this approach ignores how the reproductive technologies are rapidly transforming public health into a market for reproduction and for experimenting on the living; how within this new economy, human beings, their most intimate relations, and their descendants are becoming objects of research; how medicine itself is being used for the "industrialization of life," the management of the sexes and sexualities (Gavarini, 1990), rather than for its primary mission: to relieve or to cure. For make no mistake, many of these technologies, such as artificial insemination by donor, are far more ideological than medical in nature (Vandelac, 1988; 1989); not only are they at the frontiers of biomedicine and experimentation, they are changing radically the very meaning and the function of medicine (Vandelac, 1988; 1990a; 1992a and b).

For the most part, experts concerned with ethics, analysis and regulation have been content to examine issues raised by the NRTs *a posteriori* and case by case, not only ignoring basic questions of technological and social evaluation but also ignoring fundamental ethical questions, such as, to paraphrase Decornoy (1992:24), if human beings have the right to do by themselves and to themselves anything they want to do and everything that they can do or, more specifically, whether it is "ethical" to allow the new "industry of life" to reorganize the human being.

In a context where these questions have been largely ignored, where rigorous information and thorough analyses of practices, their objectives and their impact are few and far between, any report from the Royal Commission, even one that is biased and incomplete, even one that has little basis in original and serious research,[8] is liable to be found appealing. This is especially so if this document fits within a pre-established and hence easily digestible framework and if its recommendations to restrict certain practices and limit their "abuses" appear as easily applied "solutions." In short, if this final report from the Commission can fill the mental space long since made ready for it and if, as rumour has it, its conclusions are buried inside a thousand and one recommendations that focus attention on administrative details, people will likely reduce the indescribable history of this Commission to "simple operational problems." And if, as has also been rumoured, the report arrives in many weighty volumes, if it's prettily packaged for a November 15 launching, probably quickly pushed aside by pre-Christmas euphoria, and if it is cleverly summarized in a brief press kit, accompanied by a few images for ninety-second TV clips — how can anyone not be completely taken in?

"ACCESS" AND "FREEDOM OF CHOICE" TO REPRODUCTIVE SERVICES OR THE ART OF DIVERTING ATTENTION

From the early days of this Commission, Dr. Baird discussed the reproductive technologies in broad terms of so-called individual "choices" and of means of access to them,[9] referring to these (wrongly) as "therapeutic" and associating them with "medical services," as if the conception of a human being were of the same order as a "service," medical or not. This focus on access established the initial framework for debate.

As has been shown elsewhere (Vandelac, 1988a; 1988c; 1990b) through words and the structure of arguments, through rhetoric, that discourse insinuates the reproductive technologies into the minds of one a into the collective unconscious. Thus, the words chosen, the arguments a determine how these technologies become part of the social fabric. Wh   we examine this discourse we find that a number of terms, like nested Russian dolls, have helped to mask the different levels of reality and of what is at stake, while playing a genuine advertising role. This is true notably of the expressions "surrogate mother" (Vandelac, 1987; 1988), "pre-embryos," "surplus embryos," "fetal reduction," and numerous acronyms such as VIP, GIFT[10] or terms like "LIFE Doctor" from the "LIFE Clinic" in Toronto. In this brave new linguistic world, a term like "sterility," too often incorrectly applied to any difficulty in conceiving, gets used to dramatize the incidence of fertility problems. Similarly, the notion of "success rate" used to assess fertilization and artificial insemination programs — an elastic notion par excellence — hides the 90 percent failure rate of IVF. Similarly, too, with the word "access."

In the rhetoric of "access" and "free choice" with respect to what are called "fertility services" or, to borrow the term used in France, "medically assisted procreation" services, we find further masks. But the terms "access" and "choice" are not just camouflage. They also play a genuine role as a "locomotive" for these activities. In fact, they give the explicit impression that there is a train with a conductor, tracks — and a direction. Hearing or reading these "locomotive words," we no longer ask why or how the train — the services — started up, who or what is driving, what it contains, or where it is going. Most people, in fact, don't even notice its passage. To others, the idea of stopping this (runaway) train or of slowing it down seems impossible. The train is part of the landscape now and the only debate is about who will get on board (access) and how (free choice). At times, public protests force the removal of some cars loaded with dangerous products — which aren't always the most explosive ones — or lead to the revision of certain regulations. But the train keeps chugging along regardless.

In other words, when the talk is centered primarily about access, it means that use of the technologies is already taken for granted and implies that they are scientifically tested, ethically legitimate and socially acceptable. By focusing the debate on modes of access, matters of effectiveness, safety and long-term effects become secondary, and, even more worrying, whether these technologies are truly relevant for treating the problem is not even asked.

Yet, despite the initial emphasis of the Commission on it, access is the least of the problems, if it is one at all, with the NRTs. For example, despite photos of smiling babies and delighted parents offered as "proof" of the relevance, appropriateness and effectiveness of IVF, this technology is not very effective, still experimental and quite costly, especially within a public health context. The technologies also entail numerous risks, side-effects and iatrogenic effects (Duelli, Klein and Rowland 1988), as well as perverse social consequences including their indirect contribution to the social production of infertility (Vandelac, 1988). To reduce the debate to "access" is to camouflage all these.

Take, for example, ovulation induction by drugs, a central component of IVF often used as well in programs of artificial insemination and for women on waiting lists for diagnostic tests for infertility to force the simultaneous production of a number of mature ova. The pharmaceutical drugs used cause numerous (side) effects[11] including ectopic pregnancies (5.2 to 7 percent), which may lead to sterility; multiple pregnancies (22 to 25 times more than normal), with often heavy and sometimes tragic consequences for women, their children, and the family as a whole (see chapter by Sky); and tubal lesions, endometriosis, ovulation problems, ovarian cysts, and a higher rate of spontaneous abortions (see Laborie, 1992a and b, and St. Clair Stephenson 1992 for a documented review of the literature on these and other consequences). Is insuring access to these drugs the first priority?

This question gains relevance when we realize that even the consequences identified to date were "accidental" findings. As John Jarrell found when he reviewed 4400 manuscripts, "virtually none of these dealt with the adverse health outcomes as a primary outcome of interest.... The adverse health outcomes were all secondary." He adds: "I don't think we've done our homework very well in setting the kinds of outcome-based follow-up for some fairly severe outcomes. For example we do not know the incidence of iatrogenic infertility. That is, cases in which patients sought therapy for their infertility and were actually made worse as a consequence" (SOGC 1993:310).

Focusing attention on access blocks consideration of these issues. It also means creating a potential clientele for these technologies. Interestingly, it further implies that "access" to these technologies may be refused — and refused for reasons of moral principles or certain social norms — leading thereby to stormy debates on "freedom of choice" and individual "rights" that reinforce the notion that the technologies are a priori good and diffused for strictly "medical" reasons.

Given this confusion of the issues and their implications fostered by Dr. Baird, it is not surprising that so many of those who intervened at the public hearings to voice their concerns and to criticize this biomedical drift nonetheless concluded, through a strange twist of logic, that everyone should have access to them — with no "discrimination!"

Posing the problem in terms of access also leaves the impression that certain persons are opposed to others' wanting to have children in a way that allies clienteles with the biomedical world and lets them become media foils par excellence.[12] It also reverses the relationship of supply and demand as well as the order of responsibilities: the spread of these technologies is presented as doctors' responses to individual demands as if the shattering of maternity (De Vilaine, 1986; 1990), the marketing of sperm and ova, or the overproduction of embryos were merely "personal choices" modulated by "adequate information" and "enlightened consent."[13]

Finally, because the question of access is presented in a global manner to a public that often equates the various reproductive and genetic practices with "test-tube babies" alone, everything gets tangled together and, for example, the eugenicist motives underlying the use of pre-implantation diagnosis and selection to genetically sort embryos or the financial interests that motivate genetic experiments are silenced. This contributes, as well, to making any criticism appear as anti-medicine, anti-technology, even anti-democratic — a product of those lacking respect for individual rights or who are insensitive to the tragedy of infertile couples. What could be better than this packaging to arouse guilt about one's own reservations? And what better way to divide women's groups (all of whom are generally concerned about the "industrialization of reproduction") between those who support the rhetoric of "freedom of choice" and those who criticize this legacy of the abortion struggle as inappropriate for analysing reproductive technologies?

In sum, focusing the debate on individuals' access to artificial conception services avoids questioning the role of the medical profession in the premature, unbridled diffusion of these technologies, as well as in the inflation of so-called medical "indications" and hence of clienteles who thereby gain "access." While certain normative reasons for excluding possible clienteles are debatable, no doubt the constant widening of clienteles for reasons that have so little to do with "medicine" is even more so. Focusing the debate on questions of access as Dr. Baird did at first contributes to stimulating demand while at the same time it imposes the weight of experimentation and of its biomedical and social consequences on individuals who, by giving so-called "enlightened consent," clear the principal investigators of any responsibility for the diffusion or effects of the technologies. Above all, this analytic viewpoint and its often deceptive "therapeutic" wrapping result in doing away with any epistemological questioning of the meaning, scope and impact of this veritable "high speed rail" (TGV in French) for the transformation of the living, or of its clouded horizons and our weighty responsibilities towards future generations. With talk of "access," we content ourselves with talking about details such as the location of level crossings while the train speeds by.

ABUSES BY CERTAIN PRACTITIONERS AND THE EXPERIMENTAL NATURE OF CERTAIN PRACTICES

The April 1993 conference with which this chapter began marked a strategic turning point in Dr. Baird's discourse. For reasons of credibility and political skill, she could no longer limit herself to the rhetoric of choice and access, supporting the bulk of the practices while merely adjusting some of the modalities. The controversies over her chairmanship were too numerous, the denunciations by the academic world of Commission research for its absence of transparency and disregard for the usual rules of scholarship too virulent, and the opposition of women's groups, notably the National Action Committee on the Status of Women (NAC), too obvious. Dr. Baird was consequently forced to modify her stance to remove herself — at least in appearance — from the pharmaceutical and biomedical worlds. And this is what she did in the winter of 1993. The first occasion was during a luncheon address in Toronto, at which she began to point out certain problematical practices in reproductive technology and criticized the motives of the pharmaceutical firm Serono (major producer of fertility drugs) for funding a national register of data on IVF — funding judged liable to compromise the credibility of such a register. But the *pièce de résistance* was the press conference in April on the results of the Commission-supported investigation of "fertility programs" in Canada[14] given jointly with commissioner Bartha Knoppers. Despite the gaps in this study, these results showed overwhelmingly the haphazard nature, lack of rigour and elastic ethics of many "fertility programs."

While the press release acknowledged some of these problems, its first page devoted two paragraphs to the risk of AIDS contamination during insemination with untested fresh sperm. Following closely revelations of the tainted blood scandal,[15] this bait was too attractive for the parliamentary press not to bite! They had their headline! So much so that the paucity of the entire report and the other serious problems of Canadian practices in the field of artificial reproduction were temporarily pushed aside.

Was this a calculated gesture? The July 1993 Commission Update suggests it was. One thing is certain: the press bit a little too hard! Both Dr. Baird and her commission were tarnished (as was the federal Minister of Health whose policies were shown to be more rigorous for animal than for human insemination). Some journalists were able, in just a few days and with no resources, to conduct a more meaningful investigation of several aspects of the question than had the Commission itself. And the directors of a number of artificial conception services reacted sharply to Dr. Baird's remarks. They described the report as alarmist and, by claiming it was liable to sully the reputation of their centres, they thereby used the occasion to bolster their own services.

Once again, this rough handling by the press did not prevent Dr. Baird from getting most of her message across: Yes, there were "inconsistencies on the part of" a few "delinquent" physicians, as well as "variations in practices, data collection, record keeping and outcomes" (to use her euphemistic expression). But the findings, according to her, reflected the impressive investigative work accomplished by the Commission and justified, in advance, proposing guidelines for the so-called "fertility programs" so that, she claimed, they could provide better services.

A STRANGE COINCIDENCE

One may of course wonder why Dr. Baird waited until April to make public the study she'd had in hand for months, and why she presented it essentially in terms of "variations in practices and non-respect for the guidelines in the area" — variations that explain why certain treatments are not in "the best interests of infertile women and couples in Canada."

Whether coincidental or deliberate, this survey by the Commission was made public at the same time as the release of "Ethical considerations on the new reproductive technologies" dealing with "Banking and handling of gametes and embryos" (SOGC, April, 1993: 316-323), by the Society of Obstetricians and Gynaecologists of Canada. It is interesting to note that the point of departure for the SOGC document was the same as for the Commission's press release: the risks of AIDS transmission associated with the use of fresh sperm for artificial insemination (AI).

To what extent do the proposals by the SOGC complement the Commission's "revelations?" Or is it the reverse? One shows that services are not always "impeccable," while the other has already worked out solutions.[16]

The Commission's supposed "survey" of "fertility programs" is basically a slapdash and scientifically unacceptable work insofar as it gives no information even about such things as the number of attempted inseminations, the proportion of inseminations using the spouse's sperm compared with those using donor sperm, the frequency of use of drugs for ovulation induction or, of course, success rates. While it is known from the existing international literature that artificial insemination, essentially a G-string operation more ideological than medical (Vandelac, 1988a and b; 1989b), is inefficient and entails numerous perverse effects both individual and social, such considerations are ignored, with only the irresponsibility of certain practitioners and the failure of professional bodies to provide strict guidelines noted. In its turn, and using a public health logic that escapes us, the SOGC proposes only to speed up the diffusion and to finance the development of AI programs.

The SOGC's line of argument is very astute: given the risks of contamination by fresh "donor" sperm during artificial insemination, their use cannot be admitted.

However, given the higher costs for the use of frozen sperm in some provinces, "the Committee considers that it is urgent to sensitize provincial ministers of health to this problem and to obtain from them adequate funding for therapeutic (sic!) insemination by donor (TDI) with frozen sperm or for the use of a powerful method of detection such as polymerase chain reaction." And the panic over the risks of contaminated sperm could not have done a better job of "sensitizing" the ministers.

Continuing with the SOGC document, we read that "The CSFA and the SOGC recommend the establishment of sperm banks" that "must be assured of adequate financing to provide both impeccable service and research and development for technological improvement." They suggest, in other words, that if the services aren't always "high quality," it's because of inadequate funding, particularly for research and development! Thus, not only are the funding of frozen sperm banks and the "sensitizing" of provincial health ministers recommended explicitly, but privatization of this practice if public funding is inadequate is encouraged implicitly.

But there is more to the SOGC's "ethical" considerations. After advocating public funding for regional artificial insemination centres so that research and development can go on, the SOGC notes the need to determine "the use of frozen gametes and embryos." Note the shift in level. Using AIDS as the pretext for increasing both public funding and the development of research, the SOGC has moved directly from sperm to oocytes and embryos, lumping embryos, sperm and oocytes all together as "biological material" and asking only who should determine their use: both parents, one parent, or the centre?

The response of the SOGC to its own concern is suspicious. The donor or the parents are to specify the uses to which their frozen gametes or embryos are exclusively reserved, but if the parents have not contacted the centre for more than two years, the power to decide the fate of the frozen gametes or embryos reverts to the facility. Such singleness of purpose guarantees material for "research and development." And this purpose is underlined by the last of the SOGC's so-called ethical considerations in this specific document: "The CSFA and the SOGC endorse the use of human gametes for research investigations which have the potential to benefit individual or social needs." Each word here is a veritable rhetorical pearl. The phrase "have the potential to benefit" throws the doors wide open, because in research, everything is possible and "needs," whether general or particular, may be very broad. In other words, if everything is technically possible, everything must be done and everything must be allowed.

The document goes on: "Research on the human pre-embryo may be permissible in some circumstances, when after thorough ethical consideration there is compelling evidence that such investigations may provide significant and recognizable potential for generating new knowledge not otherwise obtainable — for benefiting human health." Notice the wording "may provide" and "not otherwise attainable" as well as the magic relation between "new knowledge" and "for benefiting human health." Again, if it is possible, it can be permitted — if there is "ethical consideration."

But can there be real ethical consideration or only its guise? Given the commitments to research and the fierce competition among scientists in this area, the SOGC recommendation for a "special committee formed of lay people, medical professionals and other scientists to monitor all such activities... in accordance with guidelines established by the Medical Research Council of Canada" is unlikely to provide reassuring ethical review.

Already, available "data show poor compliance [to existing guidelines] by many practitioners and clinics" as Dr. Baird herself acknowledged at the April press conference (RCNRT, 1993a). It would be naive to expect better adherence to new ones. But this discourse of review and control provides rich terrain for the Royal Commission's switch in emphasis from access to excess. As well, by accentuating the "poor compliance" of a few physicians and by emphasizing how certain treatments are contrary to the interests of women and infertile couples, in short by shifting from "access" to "excess" to tackle the "abuses" by certain practitioners, the Commission, with SOGC support, has also slid smoothly, but far more subtly, from medicine to experimentation.

A POLICY SHIFT BY THE BAIRD COMMISSION — OR A STRATEGIC MIRAGE?

This intriguing shift from medicine to experimentation raises several questions. One is, will the Commission follow its own lead and go so far as to admit that in vitro fertilization, for example, is a practice that has not yet been scientifically validated, signifying that it is still experimental?[17] Or will it say merely that there is "inappropriate use" of these technologies — a vague formulation that supports the technologies themselves and questions only their excessive or uncontrolled use? To admit the experimental nature of the reproductive technologies would constitute a repudiation of the authorities that have endorsed the laissez-faire policies regarding their use to now (Vandelac, 1992a). But would it lead further, to an analysis of the role played by these bodies, their premises and their mode of operation? Would it then be possible to change the focus so that women and children would no longer be the objects of experiments that are sometimes so ill-considered?[18] Would it call into question some of these practices in terms of more coherent public health priorities? Would others join the few scientists who have already recognized the improvisation and relentless pursuit that has marked this sector and would research into these experiments called reproductive technologies begin?

Regrettably, this is all unlikely and we should have no illusions about the true meaning and implications of recognition of the experimental nature of certain practices by the Commission or the SOGC. For several reasons, excess may be an even more dangerous framework for the NRTs than access.

EXPERIMENTAL? THEN LET'S EXPERIMENT — AND FINANCE THE EXPERIMENTS...

First of all, labeling the technologies experimental paradoxically opens more doors than it closes for their financial support. In the current context of cost-cutting in public health, governments cannot increase direct funding for costly technologies whose effectiveness and safety are not scientifically validated. But difficult as it may be to justify increased public funding for such unproven services, it is easy to do so under the cover of research. Thus, to admit that use of these technologies is inappropriate, or that they are not scientifically validated, is to pave the way to allocate funds for them in order to assess their appropriateness and to measure their effects.

For example, in the four years of its mandate and despite the fact that there are only "41 fertility programs," including 17 IVF programs,[19] the Commission has clearly been unsuccessful at drawing a genuine portrait of ongoing practices. Thus, the "need" for a meaningful summary of their current status could justify funding research to do just this. Following this logic, what would seem likely to be proposed, five or ten years after other industrialized nations have already done so, is the establishment of a national data register whose costs would no doubt be assumed by supervisory bodies or specific research funds. As well, and with the same logic, one could also justify the need for "regional" centres, because only these would have enough clients and enough human, financial and technical resources to permit the evaluation of the chief medical, psychological or social aspects of these practices being called for. Similarly, one could also justify increasing the research funds awarded by the numerous grant-giving bodies in this field[20] to insure levels of use of the technologies sufficient to support their analyses.

In sum, the pathetic state of practices and the extremely perfunctory nature of the Commission's inquiry seem likely to lead, paradoxically, to funding these programs in order to enable the research required by calling them experimental. And, while the side effects and risks associated with these practices should logically be an incentive to slow down or even stop certain practices, these become, instead, reasons to stimulate research, expand activities, and accelerate the growing ascendancy of technology over the reproductive process. In so doing, Canada could present an image of "responsible use of technology," while improving its weak "performances" and remaining a location of choice for research — and for the pharmaceutical industry.

It would be unacceptable if the Baird Commission used the absence of scientific validation for certain practices as a pretext to maintain or even enlarge them, claiming to do so in order to measure and improve their effectiveness and innocuousness. This would raise serious concerns about its public health priorities and its concept of "ethics."

SOCIAL AND PSYCHOLOGICAL EXPERIMENTATION

A second reason for concern about an official Commission view of these technologies as "experimental" is the likelihood that the analyses generated will focus only on the simplest and most simplistic dimensions of their consequences. The impact of reproductive technologies is in no way limited to problems about their effectiveness or harmlessness, the probable focus of "official" research. Rather, their impact is on the entire being, the whole of society. The individuals involved cannot be studied as merely "biological entities," but must be approached as individual subjects endowed with imagination and intentionality, adults inscribed in the tangles of relationships and genealogy, who may or may not repeat, in their turn, the loop of transmission. Profound social and cultural meanings and complex relationships of childbearing are affected by these technologies and require thoughtful analyses.

Already, the widespread diffusion of the technologies has given rise to mass social psychological experimentation whose breadth and effects we are barely beginning to measure.[21] As shown elsewhere (Vandelac, 1992b; 1990c; 1991), not only have the notions and the reality of maternity and paternity been turned upside down[22] but the very identity of human beings as well as our notions of sexuality, childbearing, procreation and genealogy have also been touched, transformed and sometimes even fragmented. When two or three so-called surplus embryos or fetuses are eliminated *in utero*, when women are paid to produce embryos, when proposals are made to use ovaries from fetuses for possible pregnancies of menopausal women or when young "sperm vendor" students are turned into amnesiac studs, is there not already "psychological experimentation" and "social experimentation" run amok?

As a result, even if we were able through experimentation to reduce failure rates or to limit some of the physical risks, this would still not let us legitimize either the excessive "medicalization" of conception deriving from these technologies or the questionable specific practices (e.g., oocyte maturation, genetic manipulations) which are able to transform individual human beings, even the species. And merely calling these practices "experimental" is not obviously likely to generate studies of their radical transformation of our way of conceiving human beings, though it is likely to provide justification for simplistic studies in which the practices are reduced to a narrow consumerist perspective or to simple questions of "health."

SUPPORT FOR THE RESPONSIBLE AUTHORITIES?

There is a third reason to fear a belated recognition of the experimental nature of certain practices. Unless there is rigorous analysis of their hasty, uncontrolled diffusion, backed up by a thorough examination of how they have already obtained support from ethical and evaluative authorities, the key role already played by these authorities in legitimizing their use will be "overlooked," and the premises and modalities of contemporary ethical and scientific evaluations and the responsibilities of public bodies will be left unchallenged. Are the ethical, evaluative, professional and governmental authorities who have already approved the activities now said to be problematic by the Commission credible agents to establish guidelines for this next phase of experimentation?

With few exceptions,[23] and most surprisingly, the vast majority of authorities analysing these technologies to date have evaded or altogether ignored examining their experimental nature (Trépanier, 1993). It's as if, appalled by the scope of the questions raised and trapped by the urgent need to react to a series of *faits accomplis*, these authorities had overlooked the simplest, most basic and fundamental matters, notably those concerned with experimenting on human subjects — matters that have been central to contemporary ethical reflection since the Nuremberg trials for crimes against humanity (Vandelac, 1992b).

Thus, while scientific evaluation of the technologies should be an essential component of any ethical examination, and while social evaluations should be corollaries to any scientific evaluation, existing analyses of reproductive technologies have obviously shunned rigorous ethical, scientific and social evaluation. And, it is probable that when authority for review will remain with the same individuals and groups that have had this role until now, the mechanisms of both ethical and scientific evaluation will continue to ignore social evaluations of these activities once they are (re)named experiments.

CONCLUSION

Whether the debate on reproductive technologies is framed in terms of "access" or "excess," it remains assumed that the issues are primarily medical matters of health (care). Moreover, whether seen as "access" or "excess," the discourse appears to lead to broadening the practices, at least to speeding up experiments. And by confining the debate within the narrow area of health care consumption, and claiming to want to control access or control dangerous excesses, there is a great risk that the Commission will seduce the press and reassure the public that those with power on these matters in society are finally assuming their responsibilities.

We can rejoice, of course, if these practices become more controlled. But this dodges the main issue. Drowning in the rhetoric of "health care consumption," how are we to understand that it is really whole segments of our symbolic world and of our culture — the sense of kinship, the notions of the individual and her relationships with others, the representations of time and of the body — that are shattered by these technologies? And how are we to come to a realization that the practice of medicine is being transformed from one that provides care into a biotechnical enterprise for "manufacturing" potential human beings, which has unprecedented economic, political and epistemological implications?

The reproductive technologies and their by-products, notably genetic experimentation on embryos, open new horizons that are profoundly transforming the nature, the goals and the function of medicine, changing it from "repairing" to "reproducing." Thus, our concern is not so much with medically assisted procreation as with medicine being assisted by the current transformation of procreation into a techno-economic operation for manufacturing potential humans.

These technologies take their place in a vast economic-techno-scientific complex wherein they obey perfectly the dynamic of "Science-Push" or, more precisely, the economic imperatives of techno-science. And as is characteristic of so many technological innovations, commercialization quickly follows production. As other "goods and services," the reproductive technologies can find a market only after there is a demand for them, a demand that can only be fully expressed following an orchestrated process of social legitimization which makes the demand justifiable, which makes it a new "need" (Vandelac, 1990b), and which makes us believe that different authorities — ethical and other — have for the most part endorsed them.

As we have seen, however, there has not been adequate questioning of their nature, validity and relevance, of their impact and profound meaning. In this

269

vacuum, the debate on these technologies has drifted, focusing mostly on the modes to manage them. This has helped to insure the social legitimization of their development. And, while the mandate and interdisciplinary composition of the Commission should theoretically have allowed it to fill the vacuum meaningfully, the process and structure imposed by Dr. Baird compromised this potential (See Eichler).

It is important now for the public debate to move away from legitimizing and administrative issues and toward understanding the genesis and the ideological bedrock of this technologized mutation of childbearing, and of the entrenched economic and sociopolitical interests promoting it. Interrogation of the meaning and purposes of this mutation of childbearing is fundamental and urgent. Not only are medicine, society and its ethics being transformed through these technologies, but humans and humanity are being redefined.

BIBLIOGRAPHY

For Bibliography, please see Bibliography after my article in Volume 2.

NOTES

This article is based in part on two of my research projects, "Éthique et expérimentation biomédicale sur l'être humain: les femmes et la fécondation extra-corporelle," and "Technologies de procréation: éthique biomédicale, médias et démocratie," both financed by the Social Sciences and Humanities Research Council of Canada, and carried out with research assistants, Isabelle Trépanier and Rosanna Baraldi for the first, and Rosanna Baraldi and Carolle Roy for the second. It is also based on an analysis of research contracts commissioned by the Baird Commission carried out with Gwynne Basen and presented last February at the National Association of Women and the Law Congress in Vancouver. This article also refers to many of my earlier articles cited in the bibliography, which explains why I have reduced references to the minimum here so as to confine myself to the main part of the argument. I wish to thank research assistant Évelyne Fortin as well as Andrée-Lise Méthot for their support, and also Christine Bernard-Milot, Line Lapierre and Theresa Gray for their much appreciated secretarial help. I am very grateful to Sheila Fischman for taking on with great professionalism the translation of this text. I would like to thank Gwynne Basen for her support and patience, her insightful investigative work and her deep solidarity. A special thanks also to Abby Lippman for her highly stimulating critical sense, her great generosity and her exceptional editorial skills. Finally, this text would never have been written without the leadership and the extraordinary effort of Margrit Eichler whose profound commitment to the need for a democratic process to examine the situation of NRTs in Canada led first to the creation of the Baird Commission and then to the critique and analysis of its failure. She has been an unfailing source of personal support and intellectual stimulation.

1   Taken from "The Laws of Life. Another Development and the New Biotechnologies," *Development Dialogue*, no 1-2, 1988, Dag Hammarskjold Foundation, Uppsala, Sweden. Cited in De Cortnoy, 1992.

2   Accompanied by numerous articles as well as highly critical editorials, notably in the *Gazette* and *La Presse* July 8, 1993.

3   It is surprising that there has been no genuine journalistic investigation of the hidden side of this Commission and of the consequences of such an absence of collegiality and openness especially when the consequences can lead to such fundamental transformations of human conception and of the human being itself.

4   Some 54 percent of the members of the Warnock Commission (England, 1984) came from the medical sector; the proportion was 57 percent in the Benda Report (Germany, 1985); while the report of "The Five Sages" published in France in 1986 brought together five people, including two biologists directly involved in IVF and AI, one physician and two lawyers (Trépanier, 1993). As well, the role of lobbies and the biomedical world in adoption of the English law, The Human Fertilisation and Embryology Act of 1990, testify to the impressive power of biomedicine on such authorities. On this subject, see the article by Bolton, Osborne and Cervantes (1992) on their involvement in the passage of the law.

5   This is the case in U.S. with the report of the U.S. Office of Technology Assessment and seems to be the case as well for the Wyden Report. See also Rutnam 1990 on the Australian situation.

6   For example, the report on Fertility programs in Canada, which was supposed to be one of the major tools to inform the public about the Canadian situation, gives a picture of reality that is not only incomplete but almost totally unusable because of the way in which this research was designed, carried out and presented.

7   Taken from the title of the most recent book on reproductive technologies by Robyn Rowland, this expression refers to both women and embryos.

8   Without calling into question all the research contracts carried out by this Commission, whose relevance and validity we will be able to judge only after the publication of the report, we have nonetheless been struck to see certain research contracts awarded, for example, to collect in one week "opinions of economic leaders on the subject," or to perform in a few weeks, "an analysis of techno-science and its stakes," etc. See the chapter by Eichler.

    The manipulation of the commissioners regarding the process of revising research projects, the famous "review of proposal," as is documented at length in an affidavit presented to the Federal Court. See Statement of Claim.

9   For example, can single women or lesbians have access to AI or to IVF with donor sperm? What are the conditions for access to the services by people outside major urban centers? Should they receive financial help? What kind of information should be given to persons who go to infertility clinics ? What kind of consent forms should be signed?

10 GIFT is used to designate Gamete Intrafallopian Transfer, a variation of IVF and applied for a VIP (usually used for very important people) but in the world of IVF, for a very important pregnancy.

11 In addition, a broad review of literature on the subject carried out by Françoise Laborie (1992), listed the side-effects of ovulation inducers as: weight gain: 55%; asthenia: 40%; pelvic pain: 31%; abdominal distention: 25%; nausea: 11%; hot flushes: 10 to 19%; vertigo: 10%; painful abdominal distention: 5.5%; vomiting: 5%; headaches: 1.3 to 24%; blurred vision: 1.5 to 7%; mammary discomfort: 2%.

12 A good number of IVF centres encourage forming associations of infertile couples, who often will bring pressure for the development of these practices, while laboratories such as Serono, a leading pharmaceutical company making products for ovarian stimulation, finance associations of infertile couples. The majority of IVF clinics, especially the commercial ones, also organize media events such as "IVF Babies Parties." A perfect example of an advertisement for technology appearing as "news" was an uncritical article published on the front page of *Le Devoir*, August 30, 1993 in Montreal, covering the party celebrating the one hundred IVF babies "conceived" by the Fertility Institute of Montreal, a private NRTs clinic.

13 There seems to be a growing tendency to use the notion of consent as a modality for transferring responsibility for experimentation from the researcher to the individual object of experimentation. This is obviously the logic that underlies The Baird Commission giving so many research contracts to examining the issue of informed consent.

14 It is interesting to note that the title in the English version is "A Survey of Fertility Programs in Canada" and in French is "Enquête sur les programmes d' infertilité au Canada."

15 It is estimated that 40 percent of Canadian hemophiliacs have contracted HIV from transfusions with contaminated blood.

16 In her press release, Dr. Baird took the precaution of implicitly clearing professional bodies of responsibility by emphasizing that some physicians had worked very hard to develop and promulgate guidelines, but these are rarely followed.

17 If the RCNRT admitted, for example, that IVF is experimental, it would signify that more than 25 years of experimentation on hundreds of thousands of women has been conducted outside the framework of genuine medical experimentation which includes examination of effectiveness, harmlessness, iatrogenic side effects and long-term risks.

18 For example, in France, experiments were carried out by practitioners, like Frydman, who subsequently sat on The National Ethics Committee. He was one of those responsible for such debatable experimental practices as the injection of simulated ova into the uterus of some one hundred women on waiting lists for IVF to study the problem of the expulsion of oocytes after transfer (Englert, Frydman and Testart, 1985).

19 While attempts have been made to assign blame to practitioners, we may wonder if the inadequacy of the data is attributable to the carelessness of the Commission which has obviously never taken advantage of "The Inquiry Act" which provides a mandate for investigation. The research activities of the Baird Commission were limited to only half of its four-year mandate, when in fact it would have been perfectly possible in that time framework to gather all the necessary information such as the number of times the various artificial conception techniques were used and in what fashion.

20 The Medical Research Council, The Department of Health and Welfare, The Department of Agriculture for Research on Animal Reproduction (from which these practices derive), possibly The Canadian Human Genome Project as well as many provincial research bodies.

21 As an example, while relations between men and women are fundamentally altered by these technologies, very few questions have been asked about their impact on otherness and on socio-sexual relations or on "the ethics of sexual difference," to quote Irigaray. That this aspect of the experimentation on human subjects implicit in these technologies, and that a consideration of the social relations that are at the very heart of parenthood, could be blind points in the examination conducted by the majority of authorities studyng and reporting on this area is, to say the least, not only surprising but shocking.

22 A clear example of experimentation gone out of control are certainly the gestation contracts in California where embryos from the same couple are transferred to two, three or four gestators (so-called "surrogate" mothers) at the same time. These women are legally denied the name of mother. Meanwhile gestation and delivery become second-rate undertakings for second-class women. This form of experimentation must affect how society regards maternity for all women.

23 The exceptions have been the European and American bureaus of The World Health Organization, which have denounced the uncontrolled proliferation of these technologies and the absence of rigorous medical evaluation. These criticisms have long been put forward by researchers in a number of disciplines brought together in FINRRAGE. They have also been expressed in certain Australian (Victoria) and American (OTA, 1987 and Wyden) reports.

Appendix: Statement Of Claim

Federal Court (Trial Division)

BETWEEN:

Martin Hébert, Louise Vandelac, Bruce Hatfield and Maureen McTeer

Plaintiffs

- and -

Her Majesty the Queen In Right of Canada, The Attorney General of Canada, and Patricia Baird

Defendants

STATEMENT OF CLAIM

Filed on the 6th day of December, 1991

Introduction

1. The plaintiffs are Commissioners with the Royal Commission on New Reproductive Technologies which was appointed by Order-in-Council dated October 25, 1989 and established by the federal government under the Inquiries Act R.S.C. c.I-13.

2. The plaintiff Martin Hébert is a lawyer who resides in the City of Montréal, in the Province of Québec.

3. The plaintiff Louise Vandelac is a university professor who resides in the City of Montréal, in the Province of Québec.

4. The plaintiff Bruce Hatfield is a medical doctor who resides in the City of Calgary, in the Province of Alberta.

5. The plaintiff Maureen McTeer is a lawyer who resides in the City of Aylmer, in the Province of Québec.

6. The defendant Patricia Baird is also a Commissioner and was appointed Chair of the Royal Commission. She is a university professor resident in the City of Vancouver, in the Province of British Columbia.

7. In October, 1989, the Governor in Council responded to calls from women's groups and other concerned Canadians, to broaden the discussion of the impact and control of reproductive technologies and practices beyond the medical and scientific communities, by establishing a Royal Commission, with a broad, far-reaching and important mandate.

8. On October 25, 1989 the federal government formally established the Royal Commission on New Reproductive Technologies by Order-in-Council P.C. 1989-2150...

The Mandate of the Commission and the Commissioners

9. The Order-in-Council provided that on the recommendation of the Prime Minister, the Commission was to inquire into and report on current and potential medical and scientific developments related to new reproductive technologies, considering in particular their social, ethical, health, research, legal and economic implications and the public interest and to

recommend what policies and safeguards should be applied. In particular the Royal Commission was asked to inquire into:

(a) implications of new reproductive technologies for women's reproductive health and well-being;

(b) the causes, treatment and prevention of male and female infertility;

(c) reversals of sterilization procedures, artificial insemination, in vitro fertilization, embryo transfers, prenatal screening and diagnostic techniques, genetic manipulation and therapeutic interventions to correct genetic anomalies, sex selection techniques, embryo experimentation and fetal tissue transplants;

(d) social and legal arrangements, such as surrogate children bearing, judicial interventions during gestation and birth, and "ownership" of the ova, sperm, embryos and fetal tissue;

(e) the status and rights of people using or contributing to reproductive services, such as access to procedures, "rights" to parenthood, informed consent, status of gamete donors and confidentiality, and the impact of these services on all concerned parties, particularly the children; and

(f) the economic ramifications of these technologies, such as the commercial marketing of ova, sperm and embryos, the application of patent law, and the funding of research and procedures including fertility treatment.

10. The original Order-in-Council provided for the appointment of seven commissioners: the four plaintiffs, Patricia Baird (who was also appointed to chair the Commission), Grace Jantzen and Suzanne Rozell Scorsone. Each Commissioner brought his or her own special expertise to the Commission. Together, the seven Commissioners were intended to be a truly multidisciplinary commission.

11. The individual and different fields of expertise of each Commissioner is evident from the following biographical summaries of the seven original Commissioners:

* The plaintiff Martin Hébert has been a practising lawyer in the Montréal law firm of Guy & Gilbert since May, 1989. He specializes in the field of medical and health law. From 1982 to 1987 he held a number of senior positions in the Québec government, including principal secretary to the Leader of the Opposition of the Québec National Assembly, assistant principal secretary to the Premier of Québec, principal secretary to the Québec Minister of Justice and political adviser to the Québec Minister of Health and Social Affairs. He is also a founding member and a director of the Society of Medicine and Law of Québec and sits on the ethics committees for a number of hospitals. His academic credentials include an LL.B in law from Université Laval and M.A. in medical law and bioethics from King's College in London, England.

* The defendant Patricia Baird is a professor in the Department of Medical Genetics of the University of British Columbia. She is also a member of the Medical Research Council, a member of the Science Council of Canada Study Committee on Genetic Predisposition and a member of the National Advisory Board on Science and Technology.

* The plaintiff Maureen McTeer is a lawyer and well known advocate of equality for Canadian women. She was an active member of the Canadian Coalition on Reproductive Technologies that orginially called on the federal government to establish a royal commission to study the serious legal, ethical and social problems new reproductive technologies posed for Canadian women.

* The plaintiff Louise Vandelac is an associate professor of sociology at the University of Québec in Montréal and a member of the National Bioethics Council on Research on Human Subjects. She received her Doctorate in sociology from the University of Paris and has published widely in the field of reproductive technology.

* The plaintiff Bruce Hatfield has been in private practice in internal medicine since 1959. He is currently on staff at the Foothills Hospital in Calgary, Alberta. Dr. Hatfield is an active member of many medical associations including the Canadian Medical Association Committee on Ethics, the Alberta Medical Association Committee on Ethics (which he chairs) and the Canadian Bioethics Society. He is a consultant in palliative care for Carewest and coordinator for palliative care at the Foothills Hospital.

* Grace Jantzen is currently a lecturer in philosophy of religion at the Department of Theology and Religious Studies at King's College in London, England. She is the author of many publications and articles on the philosophy of religion.

* Suzanne Rozell Scorsone is the director of the Office of the Catholic Family Life, Archdiocese of Toronto, a position she has held since 1981. She has a PhD in anthropology. She is a panellist on The Stiller Report with Vision Television and a contributor to The Catholic Register....

12. The decision of the Governor in Council to entrust this mandate to a Royal Commission with several members, from very different professional backgrounds and points of view, rather than to just one person, recognized explicitly the sensitive, moral and broad ranging nature of these complex and controversial issues to Canadian society; and the wisdom of approaching their discussion and resolution in the broadest possible forum. With so many strong people, with vastly different training, it was hoped that the final report would indeed represent an honest work of collegiality.

13. Unfortunately, from the very first meeting, the collegiality hoped for has not materialized. Instead, any attempts at collegiality have been continually undermined and over time it became apparent to the plaintiffs that all substantive decisions about every aspect of the Commission's work were being made under the authority of one person, namely the Chairperson, Patricia Baird.

14.   In fact, the plaintiffs have been progressively distanced and prevented from participating in every important decision concerning the Commission's on-going operations including the nature of the Royal Commission's research, its consultation and communication program and its organizational and financial priorities with the result that any notion of collegiality and multidisciplinarity within this Commission has been illusory.

15.   As a result of this state of affairs, existing since the beginning of our work, and now confirmed by a second Order-in-Council, the plaintiffs have been effectively denied the opportunity to participate in a full and meaningful way in all aspects of the Commission's work; and, as a result, they are unable to fulfill either their responsibility to the public or the legal mandate entrusted to them by the Governor in Council to prepare a final report.

16.   The plaintiffs believe the conduct of the Commission to date has seriously and adversely affected its work and damaged its credibility. This Commission has a budget of $25 million of public monies making it one of the costliest Royal Commissions in Canadian history. Although the plaintiffs are commissioners, they have been denied information about how and on what basis this money is being spent.

17.   Later in this claim, the plaintiffs state, in more detail, examples of the ways in which the Chairperson has effectively excluded them from effective participation in the decisions of the Commission. They also describe their attempts to resolve this impasse internally. Having, over several months, exhausted every method available to them to resolve these matters, the plaintiffs feel it is time for the Court to determine their rights and responsibilities. Short of resigning, the plaintiffs believe they have no other alternative that is consistent with their responsibilities as Commissioners.

The Second Order-in-Council

18.   From the outset this Commission has been conducted contrary to basic principles of collegiality. Far from being the joint enterprise that was intended, it quickly became a Commission dominated by the Chairperson. Despite repeated demands by the plaintiffs, to this day, no basic democratic rules concerning the conduct of meetings (such as a quorum, the adoption of the day's agenda by majority, proposals, amendments, votes, adequate drafting of minutes, and so on) have ever been respected.

19.   The plaintiffs say that this way of proceeding contravened both the spirit and the letter of the law on public inquiries; and cannot be described or defended as a mere technicality or operational matter of daily office administration, or as a difference of conflicting ideologies.

20.   The plaintiffs tried, in different ways and at different times, to have respected the mandate originally entrusted to them; and to alter this unacceptable state of affairs; sadly all attempts, in which the plaintiffs have participated to change the situation have been in vain, and the situation remains unacceptable....

21.   In the face of what the plaintiffs viewed as repeated violations of their rights and responsibilities as Commissioners and the failure, by any ordinary means, to effect a change in the situation, the plaintiffs decided, in June, 1990, to advise the government of the serious problems they faced, as well as their consequences... (They wrote a letter to Mr. Paul Tellier, requesting a meeting.)

22.   In response to the letter .... Mr. Tellier finally consented to meet with the members of the Commission in August, 1990. At this meeting all Commissionrs participated and expressed their views, with the exception of the Chairperson, the defendant Baird who was absent, without reason or notice. Mr. Tellier advised the Commissioners that the government would maintain its traditional "arm's length" relationship with this Royal Commission, and suggested the Commissioners resolve the matter internally.

23.   Shortly thereafter, however, on August 28, 1990 the Governor in Council intervened directly by issuing a Second Order-in-Council which expressly revoked crucial provisions of the original Order-in-Council and which had the effect of stripping the Commissioners of all their responsibilities (save for delivering a final report) and transferring these responsibilities to the Chairperson exclusively. Paradoxically, in the same breath, the government named two new Commissioners, Susan McCutcheon and Bartha Knoppers to help with the Commission's work. ...

24.   Under the terms of reference of the original Order-in-Council the Commissioners (that is, all seven Commissioners) were authorized to do the following:

(a) adopt such procedures and methods as they may consider expedient for the proper conduct of the inquiry and sit at such times and in such places as they may decide;

(b) rent such space and facilities as may be required for the purposes of the inquiry;

(c) engage the services of such experts and other persons as are referred to in section 11 of the *Inquiries Act;* and

(d) submit a final report.

In addition, the Commissioners were directed to file their papers and records with the Clerk of the Privy Council at the conclusion of the inquiry.

25.   Although ... these provisions were not honoured in practice by the Chairperson, at least the terms of the original Order-in-Council were faithful to and consistent with the provisions of the *Inquiries Act.* That statute specifically contemplates that where a Royal Commission is composed of more than one Commissioner, all of the Commissioners are entitled to meaningful and effective participation in the substantive work of the Commission. The second Order-in-Council substituted the authority of the Chairperson alone for that of the Commissioners in respect of matters (a), (b) and (c) listed above while at the same time leaving the Commissioners with ongoing responsibility and public accountability for the work and cost of the Commission as well as the responsibility to submit a final report. In the judgment of the plaintiffs the second Order-in-Council is entirely inconsistent with the requirements of the governing statute, the

277

Inquiries Act, and has increasingly undermined any effective and meaningful role for them in this Royal Commission. The plaintiffs say that they would never have accepted an appointment as Commissionrs under the terms prescribed in the second Order-in-Council.

26. This intervention by the Government by way of the second Order-in-Council formalized legally what had been the practice since the beginning of this Commission — and had been often denounced by the then majority of Commissioners, that is, that the Chairperson, the defendant Baird, has assumed exclusive authority to make each and every procedural and substantive decision and to exercise sole responsibility for every aspect of the Commission's work.

27. This intervention by the Government, to radically alter the respective roles and responsibilities of both the Commissioners and the Chairperson, half way through its original mandate, constitutes, to the best of the plaintiffs' knowledge, an exceptional measure, perhaps even unique, in the history of Royal Commissions of Inquiry in Canada.

28. The plaintiffs say such a situation is neither recognized by, nor compatible with the spirit and the letter of the law governing federal Royal Commissions of Inquiry, which legislation establishes a true collegiality among Commissioners serving as members on the same Commission. Indeed, such collegiality is essential to this Royal Commission which, because of the breadth and complexity of the subject matter, requires a multidisciplinary approach.

29. The plaintiffs further say that a plain reading of the federal *Inquiries Act* contemplates two types of Commissions. The first assumes one Commissioner sitting alone, in whom all authority and responsibility reside: and the second (as this Royal Commission is) assumes a larger, usually diverse or multidisciplinary group, where all powers and responsibilities are shared collectively among member Commissioners, with the Chairperson conveying to the public or the Government, as the need arises, the decisions and considered views decided by the Commissioners as a whole.

30. The immediate effect of the second Order-in-Council on this many-membered Commission, was to create, in fact, two categories of Commissioners, which is nowhere provided for in the federal *Inquiries Act.*

31. Even though the second Order-in-Council denied the plaintiffs the authority and responsibilities set out in the *Inquiries Act,* and in the original Order-in-Council and was the tool used by the Chair to formally deny the plaintiffs the opportunity, as Commissioners, to participate fully in the substantive decision making process of this Commission, the plaintiffs remain responsible for the Commission's work, publicly accountable for its expenditures and legally obligated to prepare and present a final report by the end of October, 1992.

The Alleged Breach of Confidentiality

32. The plaintiffs were and remain faced with a true dilemma — an Order-in-Council, which simultaneously made them legally responsible ... for the preparation of recommendations on a

complex and controversial area of societal concern; and yet robbed them of all resources and processes with which to accomplish that task. Now, a previously informal practice of total concentration of all authority and decision-making solely in the Chair, was incorporated into a second Order-in-Council, contrary to the spirit and the letter of the applicable legislation on public inquiries. The plaintiffs decided it was their duty to make public this unacceptable state of affairs.

33.   In separate interviews in September, 1990, three of the plaintiffs responded to questions from journalists about a number of matters involving their work as Commissioners, including their fundamentally altered responsibilities as a result of the second Order-in-Council. The result for all involved was an accusation of breach of confidentiality. Following the refusal by the Chair to produce the alleged legal opinion upon which the plaintiffs stood accused of such a breach of confidentiality, the accusation was shown to be both factually and legally false ...

34.   By relying on the second Order-in-Council, and interpreting its wording so as to give her exclusive authority over every single aspect of the Commission's work, the Chair unilaterally established a policy of confidentiality, unique to this Commission, and over and above that commitment to confidentiality to which the plaintiffs all willingly committed themselves at the beginning of their mandate. This unprecedented attempt to prevent all legitimate contact between some members of this public Royal Commission, including the plaintiffs, and members of the media covering the Commission's work, effectively confused the legitimate policy of confidentiality concerning deliberations as Commissioners, traditional to all Royal Commissions, with an imposed policy of forced silence on all questions of public interest relating to this Commission, including its conduct.

35.   In addition, this formal requirement with respect to secrecy was extraordinary for at least two other reasons. First, the Chair, the defendant Baird, demanded that each individual Commissioner acquiesce to her authority on this matter on a one on one basis; and secondly, she insisted that this be done on a differing basis. This demand by the Chair for all Commissioners to abide by her own arbitrary and unpublished rules on the matter of confidentiality, quickly led to a conflict, as futile as it was ineffective; and saw the plaintiff Vandelac, who had offered a commitment identical to that of Hébert, literally banned from participating in the Commission's meetings; in fact she was forced to resort to outside legal counsel in order to be able to resume her responsibilities under the mandate, an expense the Chair subsequently refused to compensate from Commission funds.

The Conflict of Interest Issue

36.   During this time, and relying again on the wording of the second Order-in-Council, the Chair proceeded to establish a new policy concerning acceptable outside activities, supposedly applicable to all Commissioners ...

37.   Under the guise of protecting the Commission against accusations of conflict of interest,

the Chair relied on the wording of the second Order-in-Council, and proceeded unilaterally to impose "rules" concerning potential conflict of interest situations; rules which she admitted exceeded the normal rules applicable in such situations; and which effectively limited the professional activities and opportunities of the Commissioners.

Commission Expenditures and Investigation

38.   The plaintiffs' ability to fulfill their responsibilities to prepare and present a final report will depend largely on a number of key elements, including a thorough investigation and critical analysis of the issues covered by the mandate, a professional and top-notch research program, and a wide-ranging and public consultation and communications strategy. The plaintiffs have been distanced from the definition and execution of these elements and from the decision making process concerning them as a result of the Chair's application and interpretation of the original Order-in-Council and its replacement, the second Order-in-Council of August 28, 1990.

39.   With repect to the plaintiffs' investigative responsibilities, they state they were denied the powers outlined specifically in sections 4 and 5 of Part I of the *Inquiries Act;* and confronted with decisions already taken, for instance, to carry out public opinion polls and to later make some of their results public, in spite of commitments from the Chair that these were for internal use only ... These decisions incurred incredible costs to the Commission for work whose importance and pertinence were never shown; and which, indeed, were premised on a mistaken reading of the mandate itself, which confused "public interest" with "public opinion."

40.   One of the more troubling aspects of the present situation imposed on the plaintiffs is the fact that, in spite of their inability to affect the spending of public money in any way, the Commissioners are assumed, under the applicable legislation, as well as in the minds of the public, to be responsible for the Commission's work, and therefore, logically, aware and supportive of its budgetary priorities and expenditures. Yet on several occasions, the applicants have vehemently opposed the expenditure of vast amounts of public money, unless and until these could be shown to be of direct relevance and importance to the work of the Commissioners in the preparation of the final report....

The Commission's Research Program

41.   Nowhere is the denial of the plaintiffs' role as Commissioners more problematic, given their legal responsibility under the mandate to prepare and present a final report, than with respect to the Commissioners' research program, which will not only form the backbone of this Commission's recommendations, but become one of the few real public legacies of this Commission's work. Since the beginning, the plaintiffs were never able to participate in the decision making concerning the most basic elements of the Commission's work, including most importantly:

(a) the definition of methods for recruitment and selection of the research director and team;

(b) the allocation of human, technical and financial resources for the research program;

(c) the determination of how, and under what conditions, research projects would be formulated, and to whom they would be contracted, and for what amounts; and

(d) the determination of the needs of Commissioners to carry out effective and necessary research; and to identify the expertise necessary to the drafting of the final report, including possible alternative or dissident positions or opinions.

42.   In addition, the language of the second Order-in-Council was used by the Chair to allow her to systematically refuse to provide, or allow staff members to provide, to all Commissioners, clear and complete information on the entirety of the research program. This information is indispensable to the plaintiffs' full understanding and critical analysis of the relevance of the proposed research to the issues of their mandate, and to the recommendations of the final report ....

43.   Indeed it was only in April, 1991, as a result of repeated demands by several Commissioners, that a research proposal review mechanism was finally put in place, to supposedly answer the concerns set out above.

44.   While this process was described as one establishing a true review of research proposals, such, in fact, was never the case. Indeed, at no time since then were the plaintiffs able to obtain the essential information concerning the research program (such as the cost of each research project, the identity of each researcher, the total research budget and other key elements that would have enabled the plaintiffs to better assess and understand the purpose, relevance and priorities of the research program in light of the Commissioners' needs for the preparation of the final report); nor were they able to see on a consistent basis the individual comments of most of the other Commissioners, including the Chair; nor were they provided with the opportunity to discuss and evaluate collectively with all Commissioners either the master research plan or individual research projects ... Indeed, while the plaintiffs were reviewing, in good faith, research "proposals" presented to them by the Chair, through the Research Director, many had already been worked out with, and assigned to, outside researchers, approved formally by the Chair, with many even in the process of being completed, often without the Commissioners' knowledge; and certainly without their real input, discussion or approval.

45.   Today, more than two years after the beginning of the Commission's work, and less than a year before its formal conclusion, the plaintiffs say that:

(a) there are about 50 research projects still being prepared, the tenure and pertinence of which remain unknown to them;

(b) the reasons justifying the rejection or the merging of several research projects into one have never been revealed to them;

(c) less than 30 research projects out of a total of approximately 130 have been submitted to the Commissioners for their comments as part of this research proposal review;

(d) some 15 pieces of research were submitted as manuscripts, addressed to the Commissioners, without any previous opportunity for the Commissioners to examine all aspects of the work, including the proposals and work plans; and

(e) they have yet to be told the exact process of elaboration, approval and amendment applicable to all research projects.

46.   In spite of this, the plaintiffs were very recently able to discover, quite by accident, the work plans for the Commission's research for all four working groups (two of which are included here), which had not been available to Commissioners; and which included extensive information, including the names of the researchers and their proposals, the approximate budget of each and their individual work schedules ...

47.   Furthermore, despite repeated assurances by the Chair that what was available to the Commissioners was the sum total of the research plan and projects, the plaintiffs state that the list of research projects, given to the Commissioners ... is a partial one at best; and, according to a document the plaintiffs obtained accidentally, it appears that even after the research review process was instituted in the Spring of 1991, certain other projects were authorized and begun ... without even being brought to all the Commissioners' attention; and this despite numerous undertakings by the Chair promising this would be done; and reiterated in a memorandum, dated October 17, 1991, from Sylvia Gold, the Director of Research for the Commission to the Commissioners ...

48.   These decisions to restrict, and even withhold information, crucial to the full exercise of the plaintiffs' legal mandate, were taken by the Chair as a result of her indefensible interpretation of the original Order-in-Council, and the wording of the second Order in Council ...

Consultation and Communication

49.   As with matters of investigation and research, the process imposed by the Chair on all aspects of the Commission's work extended to matters of consultation and communication, which resulted over time in the reduction of the role of the Commissioners to that of simple advisors, distanced from the substance of all decision-making about the fundamental issues at stake in the inquiry's mandate. The result of this process was to change the character of this Commission and its work.

50.   By way of example of this denial of the intended multidisciplinary approach and involvement of many professions and points of view within the Commission's membership, the plaintiffs refer to two official Commission meetings, one dealing with constitutional law, and the other with the uniformity of laws. The preparation for these meetings was held, to the best of the plaintiffs' knowledge, without the involvement of those Commissioners who are also lawyers, thereby denying them the opportunity to participate fully in the elaboration of the fundamental legal questions at stake in the Commission's mandate; this effectively denied these Commissioners any real involvement in the definition and formulation of the Commission's work, even in their own area of professional expertise.

51.   Further, in the matter of consultation and communication, the rigidity of the format adopted by the Chair, made possible by the changes enshrined in the second Order-in-Council, and imposed on Commissioners during the lengthy and no doubt costly public hearings process (although its full cost remains hidden from the plaintiffs), prevented the plaintiffs from truly pursuing the important matters raised by intervening individuals and groups, forcing them instead to resort to a limited and superficial discussion with intervenors, focusing on the form rather than the substance of the process.

52.   A series of new consultations have recently been set up and are proceeding, in spite of determined opposition from a majority of Commissioners, who decided that it was inopportune, at this late stage in the Commission's work, to devote their energies and considerable human, material and financial resources to try and overcome the gaps resulting from the inadequacy of the original consultations and public hearings process. It is clear beyond any doubt that from now on, top priority must be given to an in-depth and full discussion among Commissioners of the many and complex questions addressed to them in the Commission's mandate....

53.   Further, the assumption that Commissioners were responsible for the work of the inquiry, and therefore both aware of, and in agreement with, the activities of the Commission, was made even more difficult to refute because of the Chair's insistence that all external communications on behalf of the Commission be handled by her. These external communications were presented as the view of all Commissioners, whether or not the matter to be made public had even been discussed or considered among Commissioners within a reasonable time frame; and even, on occasion, presented by the Chair, in spite of vehement opposition by several of the Commissioners. On other occasions, this policy even extended to making public, material and findings of work whose content and execution had been hotly contested by the majority of the Commissioners and which the Chair had promised would be used for internal purposes only....

Extension of the Life of the Commission

54.   Over and above the investigative, research, consultation and communication decisions which the Chair has arrogated to herself, other substantial decisions of great consequence, both financial and organizational, were also taken by the Chair. Of these other decisions the most notable is the decision to seek a one-year extension of the Commission's original two-year mandate in spite of the fact that there had never been any formal discussion of this matter among Commissioners.

55.   Like the other Commissioners, the plaintiffs were faced with the result of a request to the Prime Minister for an extension of the term of the Commission's mandate, made by the Chair, and pretending to be on the Commission's behalf. The plaintiffs became aware of this request only after the fact, which deliberately robbed them of the opportunity to express their profound disagreement about the need for and cost of such an extension...

Conclusion

56.   In the light of all the facts set out above, along with the supporting documentation appended, it is clear that throughout the life of the Commission all matters of substance and procedure reflected the position of the Chair, while giving an erroneous public impression of both collegiality and multidisiplinarity. This process and state of affairs have effectively and increasingly denied the plaintiffs, as Commissioners, the opportunity to answer fully, if at all, for the operation of this Commission, including its decisions, orientations, work and the cost attributed to it, to the point that their attendance and participation at meetings and other official gatherings of the Commission have become less and less pertinent.

57.   This way of proceeding and operating imposed upon Commissioners unilaterally by the Chair since the beginning of their work, and enshrined in law as a result of the second Order-in-Council, denies the plaintiffs the possibility to carry out fully, if at all, the legal mandate given to them by the Governor in Council, risks potentially damaging the personal and professional reputation of all Commissioners, compromises the credibility of the work of this Commission and may ultimately contribute to the public discrediting of the institution of Royal Commissions in Canada.

58.   In spite of recent correspondence advising the appropriate authorities of their intention to proceed to Court to have these issues resolved, matters remain unchanged; and the plaintiffs are forced now to have recourse to the only option left to them in order to clarify the nature and extent of their responsibilities as Commissioners.

Relief Claimed

59.   The plaintiffs claim:

(a) a declaration that the Schedule to the second Order-in-Council P.C. 1990-1801 dated August 28, 1990 is inconsistent with and contrary to the *Inquiries Act*, R.S.C. 1985, C. I-13 and accordingly is of no force and effect;

(b) a declaration that the plaintiffs are entitled to human, technical and financial resources, from the Commission's existing budget, sufficient to enable them to prepare and submit a report in both official languages to the Governor in Council as provided for in the original Order-in-Council P.C. 1989-2150 dated October 25, 1989;

(c) a declaration that the defendant Patricia Baird, has conducted the Royal Commission on New Reproductive Technologies in a manner contrary to the provision of the *Inquiries Act*, R.S.C. 1985, c. I-13 and contrary to the provisions of the original Order-in-Council;

(d) their costs of this action; and

(e) such further and other relief as this Honourable Court may deem just.

DATED at Toronto, this 6th day of December, 1991.

ABOUT THE AUTHORS

Maria Barile has been a disability rights activist since the early 1970s. She is one of the founders of DAWN Canada and DAWN Montreal (DisAbled Women's Network). She recently received a masters degree in social work and plans to do research and policy analysis on women and disability issues.

Gwynne Basen is a writer and film maker. She is the director of *On the Eighth Day: Perfecting Mother Nature,* a series of two films on the new reproductive and genetic technologies, co-produced and distributed by The National Film Board of Canada. She also co-produced, *I Lease Wombs, I Don't Sell Babies,* a video tape on the subject of preconception agreements, distributed by Cinéma Libre, Montreal. She is currently co-chair of the Reproductive Technologies Committee of The National Action Committee on The Status of Women (NAC). She lives in Montreal with her husband and two children.

Annette Burfoot teaches feminism, and the sociology of science and technology at Queen's University. She is also the Managing Editor of the *Encyclopedia of Reproductive Technologies* (New York: Garland Pubs., 1996).

Varda Burstyn is a Toronto based writer who was born in Israel in 1948. She has written extensively on the social and political implications of ideologies and practices involving the body — from issues of pornography and censorship, to medicine and sport. From 1990 to 1992, she was co-chair of the Health and Reproductive Technologies Committee of The National Action Committee on The Status of Women (NAC), and the principal author of its brief to the Royal Commission on New Reproductive Technologies. She is completing a book on sport, gender and politics.

Gena Corea, born in 1946, became an investigative reporter in 1971 and her articles have appeared in such publications as The *New York Times, Ms., Commonwealth, The Progressive, Omni,* and *Mother Jones* and in many anthologies published in the United States, Britain, Germany, France and Australia. She is the author of *The Hidden Malpractice: How American Medicine Mistreats Women* and *The Mother Machine: Reproductive Technologies from Artificial Insemination to the Artificial Womb.* She is the co-founder of the Feminist

International Network of Resistance to Reproductive and Genetic Engineering (FINRRAGE), and its journal and she is now associate director of the Institute on Women and Technology.

Margrit Eichler is a professor of Sociology at the Ontario Institute for Studies in Education (OISE). She has been following the NRGTs since the first case of a preconception arrangement in Canada in 1982. Her books include *The Double Standard* (1980), *Families in Canada Today* (1988) *Nonsexist Research Methods* (1988).

Lynn Glazier is a journalist and radio documentary maker living in Montreal. She is a regular contributor to Centrepoint on CBC Radio's national current affairs program *Sunday Morning,* and has won national and international awards for her documentary work in the area of health reporting. She began her career 12 years ago, working with CBC television and radio in Calgary, Toronto and Montreal, and is a native of Oshawa, Ontario. Her chapter in this book is based on several months of extensive research for her Centrepoint documentary "Playing God: Medical Ethics and History's Forgotten Lessons."

Sandra A. Goundry is a legal consultant and researcher specializing in human rights and Charter issues. She was commissioned by CDRC to prepare their original brief to the Royal Commission on New Reproductive Technologies.

Abby Lippman is based in the Department of Epidemiology & Biostatistics at McGill University and is Chair of the Human Genetics Committee of the Council for Responsible Genetics. Her research focuses on the application of genetics from a feminist perspective, emphasizing the increasing geneticization of health and illness and the biopolitics of biomedicine. She and her two children have lived in Montreal for the past 20 years, but her Brooklyn-accented French immediately reveals her New York City origins.

Christine Massey is a graduate student in the Department of Communication, Simon Fraser University and a researcher at the Centre for Policy Research on Science and Technology. Her research examines decision-making on issues of science and technology.

Judy Rebick was the President of The National Action Committee on the Status of Women from 1990-1993. She was the spokesperson for the Ontario Coalition for Abortion Clinics from 1981-1987.

Sunera Thobani is currently President of The National Action Committee on the Status of Women (NAC). As a member of the India Mahila Association, she helped organize against the opening of sex selection clinics in B.C. She is also a founding member of SAWAN (South Asian Women's Action Network) and worked toward the opening of a South Asian Women's Centre in Vancouver. She has written and spoken on the new reproductive technologies, violence against women, racism and multiculturalism, women of colour and the feminist movement, and colonialism and nationalism. She was born in Bukoba, Tanzania, and is now a Doctoral Candidate in Sociology.

Sari Tudiver is an anthropologist by training who works as a researcher and consultant in the areas of women's health and international development. Since 1991 she has been employed at the Women's Health Clinic in Winnipeg conducting qualitative research on Manitoba women's experiences with prenatal diagnosis and working to establish a Canadian Women's Health Network. She has a particular interest in the global pharmaceutical industry and the social implications of reproductive and contraceptive technologies.

Louise Vandelac has a doctorate in sociology from the University of Paris. She is a professor in the Department of Sociology at l'Université du Québec à Montréal. She was a member of the National Council on Bioethics for Research on Human Subjects from 1988 to 1991 and a Commissioner on The Royal Commission on the New Reproductive Technologies from 1989 to 1991. She has both researched and published widely on the questions of the ethical, economic and social issues that relate to the new reproductive technologies and on the role of the media in this area.

Volume II of *Misconceptions: The Social Construction of Choice and the New Reproductive and Genetic Technologies* will follow the publication of this current volume.

It contains:

Part IV: The Construction of Infertility

Part V: Women As Gestators; Children As Products

Part VI: Public Policies,
*   National Action Committee on the Status of Women
*   Council For Responsible Genetics
*   Feminist International Network of Resistance to
    Reproductive and Genetic Engineering

You can reserve a copy in advance of printing through your bookstore or by calling Voyageur Publishing's toll free number:
1-800-268-2946.
You will be billed when the book is shipped.

As well, you can write to us at:
Voyageur Publishing/Project: Misconceptions
82 Frontenac Street, Hull, Quebec J8X 1Z5

Voyageur Publishing considers complete unsolicited manuscripts.
If you have a manuscript please address it to:
Voyageur Publishing/New Manuscripts
82 Frontenac Street, Hull, Quebec J8X 1Z5